105 WEIGHT LOSS SOLUTIONS

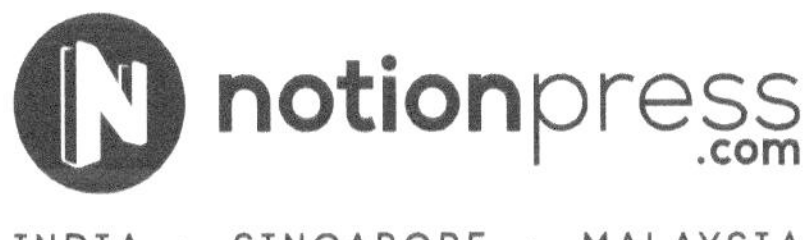

notionpress.com

INDIA • SINGAPORE • MALAYSIA

105 WEIGHT LOSS SOLUTIONS

Decoding the Secrets of Slimming, Dieting and Healthy Living

RAM GUPTA

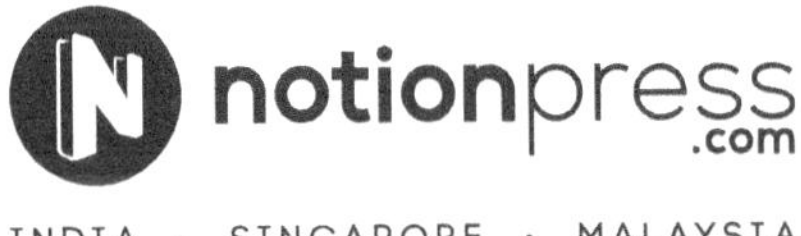

notionpress.com

INDIA • SINGAPORE • MALAYSIA

Notion Press

Old No. 38, New No. 6
McNichols Road, Chetpet
Chennai - 600 031

First Published by Notion Press 2018
Copyright © Ram Gupta 2018
All Rights Reserved.

ISBN 978-1-64249-235-4

Disclaimer

The information in this book is purely educational, and is intended to help readers be better informed when it comes to fat loss and weight management. The advice contained in this book does not take into account your individual health, medical, physical, or emotional situation or needs.

The author in not in any way engaged in providing any medical, diagnostic, or prescription advice. He has shared general advice on weight loss and it's not meant to be a substitute for the medical advice of a licensed physician.

Every attempt has been made to ensure that the information provided in the book is accurate and complete. However, the author absolves himself from any personal liability for use of information contained in the book, along with any errors, omissions, inconsistencies, or inaccuracies there may be in the content provided.

The reader is advised to consult their physician, physical fitness trainer, nutritionist, or dietician before starting a new physical exercise or diet program or making any other changes to their lifestyle.

Contents

Preface

Have you ever noticed that human beings are only species on the planet that tend to put on weight and end up with problems like morbid obesity?

That's right. No other animal, when left in its natural environment, will get unnaturally fat. Being overweight is not something that nature devised for its creatures. It's 100% man made, and it's a disease that's spreading at a rapid rate.

With increasing levels of income, people today indulge in mindless consumerism. This is especially true when it comes to food. People have stopped eating for nutrition; they now eat to appease their taste buds. And when you take into consideration the hunger and food deprivation that's ravaging the third-world, obesity becomes all the more terrifying.

As a health enthusiast, I was deeply troubled by this phenomenon. So I started reading up on the matter. And the more I read about it, the more convinced I got that staying fit should be a practice that must be cultivated by us together as a society.

Weight loss has more to do with staying healthy than losing weight for aesthetic reasons. It's medically proven that being overweight can harm your body in more ways than one. And it also takes a toll on your self-esteem and mental health.

Among children, especially, obesity cannot be tolerated. They must be taught the importance of staying healthy and being fit, because the future depends on them. And the only way to do that is parents model a healthy lifestyle to inspire their children.

With the hope of making a difference, I started writing a series of articles on weight loss. From diet to exercise to portion control to emotional wellbeing, I've covered a wide range of topics. My aim is that by the time you're done reading the book, you'll have an all-encompassing knowledge about the topic, which, in turn, will help you take a more well-rounded approach towards losing weight and keeping it off.

Weight loss is a process. *It's a journey.* And like any journey you may have undertaken, you know that it's impossible cover the entire distance in one go. You start right at the beginning, then move from one milestone to the other. Some are easier and the others a little more difficult. But you just stick it out no matter how hard it gets, because the rewards awaiting you at the end of the road are worth it.

I would like to invite you on this journey with me. Let's travel together and come on the other side with a healthier body, higher self-esteem, happier mind, and at least a couple of waist sizes smaller!

1

Top 10 Flat Belly Foods

Almost without exception, weight gain is the result of poor eating habits, an unbalanced diet, and the absence of a regular exercise routine. Certain foods, especially fried or processed foods, cause excessive fat gain in all sorts of unwelcome places, like your belly. Fortunately, there are foods which fight back against weight gain. Eaten at the right time and in the right proportions, they can accelerate your metabolism, helping you burn extra calories and reach your weight loss goals. Here are the top ten wonder foods to boost your diet plan:

Berries

Blueberries especially are the dietary equivalent of kerosene on your fat-burning fire, but other berries don't fall short either. A low-calorie favorite of seasoned diet gurus, a cup of blueberries contains only 85 calories, and the same amount of strawberries has just 52. What they contain is just as important as what they don't—not only are they packed with vitamins A, C, E, K, B6 and B12, they're full of appetite-appeasing fiber, satisfying your hunger and fighting bloat. Blue and red berries in particular (their color caused by the chemical anthocyanin) are best for getting a flat stomach, so reach for blueberries, strawberries, cherries and even red grapes at the grocery store. Adding a handful of these superfoods to your cereal, yogurt, or even your salad is a simple formula for a flat belly!

Flax Seeds or Linseed

Flax seed, also known as linseed, is full of fiber and monounsaturated fats, which are scientifically proven to aid in both breaking down body fat and lowering cholesterol. Their high fiber content aids digestion and eliminates constipation, reducing belly bloat. Simply sprinkle a spoonful into your salad or cereal or add them to your smoothie, and your pants will be fitting better before you know it!

Yogurt

The best kept secret of those slender French ladies isn't really a secret at all—it's *yogurt*. Yogurt has been an integral part of a healthy diet for Indians and the French for a long time. Rich in calcium, carbs, and proteins, it's a perfectly balanced meal or snack. But buyer beware—read those labels carefully. Some companies try to satisfy their customers' sweet tooth by filling their product with added fat and sugar.

Yogurt is a popular breakfast food for dieters, since it's both filling and low-calorie. Indians eat yogurt in a number of ways, most commonly with a glass of buttermilk at breakfast and after lunch, as it's both nutritious and hydrating. No matter how you enjoy it, yogurt is a complete, nourishing meal for fat burning, paving the way to a sexy belly.

Water and Green Tea

Water might not be food, exactly, but it's an essential part of your weight loss plan. Researchers have proven that drinking 8–10 glasses of water per day flushes toxins and reduces the water retention giving you that unsightly belly bulge for a flatter, sexier tummy. Carbonated water can make bloat worse, though, so steer clear—if you absolutely can't abide water, try green tea instead. Quite a few studies have linked green tea to accelerated metabolism, probably due to the compound catechin, which helps the body release fat from its cells and improves liver function. For best results, add 5–6 cups of green tea to your diet daily.

Cauliflower

Cauliflower might just be nature's perfect diet food. It's low in starch and calories, high in vitamins and minerals like phosphorus and vitamin K, and possibly the most versatile vegetable around. You can eat it raw in salads or dipped in your favorite low-fat dressing, steamed with some crunchy almond slivers for a filling side dish, or roasted with olive oil. Craving buffalo wings? Try dressing some steamed cauliflower with low-cal buffalo sauce. Can't make it through another weekend without pizza? Believe it or not, ground cauliflower can be made into a low-carb and low-calorie pizza crust! With only 25 calories per serving, make sure you stock your fridge and freezer with nature's most versatile vegetable.

Soups

Food connoisseurs consider soups to be appetite builders, which is why they're generally served before the meal. However, a watered vegetable broth will not only fill you before your meal, keeping you from overindulging during your main course and dessert, but will also provide you with fiber from the vegetables. A diluted soup with cabbage, spinach, cauliflower and carrots is an excellent flat tummy food. And forget the rules—soup doesn't have to be limited to lunch and dinner. It makes an excellent snack as well. Just be careful when purchasing pre-made soups—they tend to have a lot of salt, so look for the readily-available low-sodium options.

Lentils

Lentils and other beans are low in fat but rich in fiber, protein, vitamins and minerals, making them an excellent weapon in your flat-belly arsenal. Here is yet another versatile gift from nature; lentils can be steamed, cooked in gravy, roasted and salted for a healthy snack, or even sprouted and mixed in a salad. Lentils can both accompany a meal, or be the meal themselves, without adding excess calories, fat or carbohydrates to your diet.

3 Apples

An apple a day keeps the doctor away, but three apples a day banish fat! Apples are rich in insoluble fiber, so eating one before each meal helps you to eat less without compromising on nutrition. Remember—weight loss is a numbers game. Eating fewer calories than your body needs forces it to draw on those unsightly fat stores for energy, resulting in a slim, trim waistline.

Almonds

Almonds have the lowest calories of most commercially available nuts, and are both filling and nutritious, making them an excellent, convenient snacking option, especially if you choose healthier raw almonds instead of their roasted, salted counterparts. They're a powerful antidote to hunger pangs, but pay attention to the serving size—almonds pack a significant caloric punch compared to the other foods on our list, and these tasty nuts go down easy!

Salads

Fresh green salads have tremendous nutritional value. Rich in fiber, they contain practically zero calories and almost no fat. And salads are full of proteins, vitamins and minerals. You might think of salad as just a side dish, but if you're creative, they can be a full meal or even a snack. Remember to choose darker greens, as they have the highest nutritional content, and try to add as much color as possible to your salad. Not only will this make your salad as savory for your eyes as it is for your stomach, but it'll provide you with a wide range of vitamins and minerals. Cucumber, tomatoes, turnips, carrots, sprouts, bell peppers, even fruit will dress up your salad and leave you feeling satisfied. Just make sure to choose a low-fat dressing, and consider dipping your fork into a dish of dressing on the side before taking a bite, instead of drenching your greens in oil and fat.

There you have it, our top ten picks for flat-belly foods! You'll be amazed by the difference a few small changes in your diet can make on your body. Try it; after all, what do you have to lose, except weight?

2

How to Lose Weight as You Age – Four Weight Loss Secrets Revealed

Hitting a milestone birthday like 60 often comes with a fair amount of introspection and reminiscence. Your party pictures might have revealed a startling truth—you've gained some weight over the years, and if so, you're probably worried you won't be able to lose it as easily as you gained it. The fad weight loss programs, those inspirational stories with their incredible 'before and after' photos—they all feature younger people, with hardly a person over 40 to be seen. What about seniors?

The good news is that you, too, can lose weight, and you don't have to kill yourself in a marathon training program to do it.

1. Understanding Your Body's Changes

Your body isn't the same as it was a few decades ago. Your metabolism is lower, and you have less muscle mass, meaning you'll have to work harder to lose weight than you did in your 30s and 40s. That's no reason to give up before you've even started, though. You can still regain some of that muscle mass and raise your resting metabolism through exercise.

2. Exercise

Exercise doesn't have to mean sweating it out in a gym, simultaneously boring yourself and torturing your body with heavy weight repetitions and high-impact cardio. Respecting your body's capabilities and limitations is an essential part of building a sustainable exercise routine. If you push yourself so hard you're too sore to work out for several days, or worse, injure yourself, you won't be able to reach your long-term weight loss and fitness goals. Try starting with a brisk walk every other day, or a bit of light cycling. You'll still be burning extra calories and toning your muscles, and, provided your calorie consumption remains the same, you'll start losing weight. Remember, whatever your age, weight loss is only healthy when it's a gradual process as a cumulative result of healthy lifestyle changes. Even if you only lose two pounds a month, that's still excellent progress. Imagine where you'll be in six months!

3. The 'Right' Exercise

We've all heard the disclaimer, "consult your physician before beginning any exercise program," but it's more important now than ever. Your doctor can help choose the safest, healthiest program for your individual health needs.

4. Diet

Exercise is an essential part of a weight loss program, but 80% of weight loss happens in the kitchen. In other words, exercise is important, but diet is crucial. Your metabolism simply can't handle the abuse it could when you were younger, so try to remember that before you eat that soda and burger, or order that pizza at 10 p.m. on a Saturday. If you haven't already, it's time to really cut back on simple sugars, processed foods and alcohol, and embrace healthier food choices that will make you feel stronger and more energetic.

Swap out fatty red meat for high-quality lean proteins, such as egg whites, skim milk, chicken or fish, nuts, and legumes. Including a variety of fruits and vegetables in your diet will add essential vitamins and minerals, as well as helping keep your calorie count in check. Make healthy beverage choices too, such as water or home-brewed green tea instead of soda. In as little as a few days, not only will you look better, you'll *feel* better.

3

Weight Loss with Ayurveda – How It Works

Ayurveda is one of the fastest growing systems of alternate medicine, spreading quickly to the west from its origin in India. Most people associate it with massage, relaxation, and treatment of illnesses, but Ayurveda also offers weight loss solutions. Many people have adopted Ayurvedic practices for successful weight loss, and as a bonus, restored a greater sense of balance and harmony in their lives.

Understanding Ayurveda

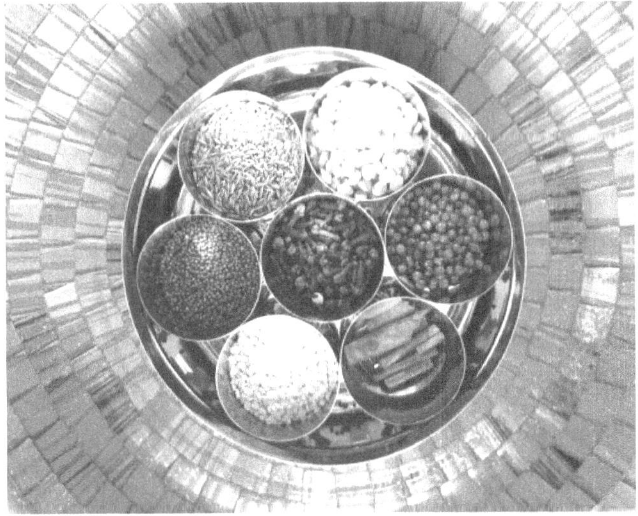

To understand how Ayurveda works for weight loss, one must first understand the system itself. According to Ayurveda, life is a process which involves the interaction of three forms of energies, or *Doshas: Vata, Pitta* and *Kapha.* These energies are present in every individual, and one can only achieve physical, mental and spiritual health when these energies are in balance. If you're struggling with obesity, or excessive stress, irritability, depression, frequent illness or other maladies, it's a sign these energies are out of balance.

Ayurveda and Weight Loss

Ayurvedic practices differ from modern weight loss tenets, which focus simply on calories in, calories out as the key to losing pounds. Rather than simply focusing a mathematical ratio as a path to weight loss, Ayurveda seeks to understand *how* and *why* your energies are out of balance. For most people, these *doshas* aren't present in equal measure; it's more likely that you identify with one or two predominant energies.

The Energies

Vata is the energy of motion and doing. It's responsible for digestion, circulation, respiration, creative thinking, emotions, and speech. People who are predominantly *vata* are easily excitable, highly energetic, and restless, and may struggle with focus and concentration.

Pitta is the fire energy. It's responsible for metabolism and intellectualism. *Pitta* people do not gain or lose weight easily; they're very sensitive to light, have a great appetite for sweets, and a high capacity to learn and concentrate.

Kapha is the energy of earth and water, controlling the organs, tissues and cells of the body. It directs joint lubrication, memory retention, and muscle and bone strength. *Kapha* individuals have strong, thick-set bodies, and are trustworthy, loyal and compassionate. Their minds are steady, but they often have a slow metabolism, making them prone to putting on weight and resistant to losing it.

Diagnosing Imbalances and Taking Corrective Measures

Imbalanced *doshas* cause physical and mental repercussions. The first thing an Ayurvedic practitioner will do is study your physical and mental characteristics, in order to identify your predominant energy or energies. Then, he'll diagnose your imbalances and prescribe lifestyle, diet and exercise changes so you can achieve a state of balance and harmony. For instance, if he finds your obesity is linked to an imbalance in your *Kapha Dosha,* he'll likely prescribe light meals, avoidance of iced drinks, oily foods, and dairy, and a flexible exercise routine.

The benefits of Ayurveda are clear, not only for weight loss, but for the pursuit of balance and harmony in all areas of your life. If other weight loss strategies haven't been working for you, perhaps it's time to give Ayurveda a try!

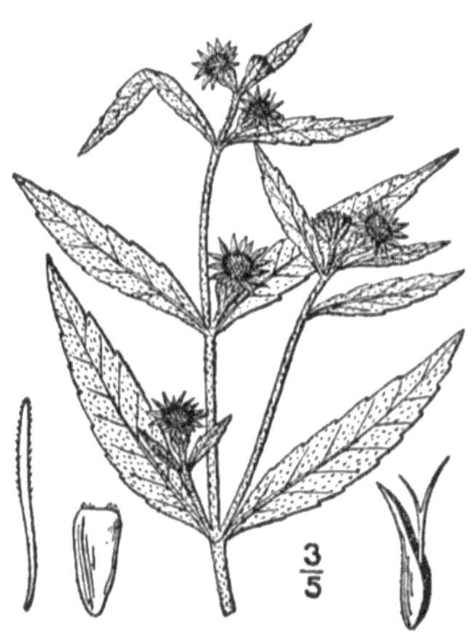

4

Want to Lose Weight Fast with Artificial Sweeteners? Think Again!

Even children know that sugar is loaded with calories and leads to weight gain. So when people begin a weight loss journey, sugar is often the first thing to go. It's not easy to give up the comfort of that first sweet sip of morning coffee or rich bite of dessert, though, so science came up with an apparent solution: artificial sweetener. All of the taste, with none of the calories? It sounds like a perfect solution. A few years ago, however, a university research team in the U.S. made a startling discovery; rather than aiding weight loss, artificial sweeteners may in fact be sabotaging it.

Artificial Sweeteners and Weight Gain

The idea might seem counterintuitive, but the reasoning is backed by solid science. The key lies in our body's metabolism. Up until recently, all sweet foods the body encountered were high in calories. As soon as your tongue tastes something sweet, your body reacts in preparation to receive and process a high-calorie meal. Core body temperature rises; the metabolism speeds up to meet the imminent digestive requirements. But artificial sweeteners don't deliver the calories their taste promised. When those calories don't turn up, your body demands more food to replace the fuel it spent in preparation. In other words, you're still hungry, and that slice of cake is looking very tempting.

If your metabolism continues to be disappointed by the empty promises of artificial sweeteners, in time it may stop reacting to the taste of sweetness, which means when real sugar and calories appear, it will be ill-prepared. Instead of burning them, your body will store them as excess fat, leading to weight gain.

Proof and Evidence

Though these studies have only been performed on rats, and not on human subjects, there is plenty of evidence available to support the theory. Obesity has already reached an unprecedented level in America, and continues to grow at an alarming rate, despite the popularity of sugar-free sweets and diet drinks. Studies have also shown that diet soda is linked to a greater risk of obesity. Though it may not yet be proven conclusively, evidence certainly seems to be pointing to some kind of link between artificial sweeteners and obesity. Sadly, it seems that there really is no shortcut to weight loss; if you want to drop pounds, the best and only path is a healthy, balanced diet and regular exercise.

Don't go racing back to sugar, though. Sugar has its own risks associated with obesity and other health problems, such as heart disease and diabetes. Use sugar seldom and sparingly, and remember that your body is probably too smart to be tricked.

5

4 Secrets to Weight Loss Workout Success

There are more weight loss and exercise programs out there than we could possibly list here, and it seems like a new one joins the list every day. So which one is the most effective? There's no easy answer to that; it all depends on your goals and personality. What really matters is your approach—taking the right steps to maximize its effectiveness. Here are four universal strategies that can help make any workout a winner.

1. Stay Hydrated

It's remarkable how many people forget this simple step. Neglecting to bring a bottle of water or sports drink with you on your workout can have some very negative consequences, both in the short term and the long.

When your body isn't hydrated, it fatigues faster and recovers slower. Your hydrated body might be able to sustain the effort of your workout for forty-five minutes, but without water, you might find yourself struggling to make thirty. That's fifteen minutes of calorie-burning you've lost due to dehydration. Your muscles are also less efficient at recovery in a dehydrated state, and less able to flush out the lactic acid buildup from your workout, causing soreness, so your next workout will suffer as well, as you try to coax your aching body into motion. Even your metabolism suffers when dehydrated. Staying hydrated is the easiest way to maximize the number of calories you burn, and your overall health in general.

2. Rest is Crucial

Don't underestimate the value of rest. As you grow stronger and start to see results, it's very tempting to skip those rest days and push yourself harder. Your body needs those days, however, to strengthen and repair your muscles. Stronger muscles burn more calories, which translates directly to weight loss. Without rest, you risk fatigue and injury, and you'll soon find yourself struggling to sustain your workouts. Make sure to schedule a rest day or two every week.

3. Words of Wisdom

"Don't do everything every day, or the same thing every day." Eventually, your body will adapt to routine, and if you don't challenge it regularly with something new and different, you'll reach a plateau. The best strategy is to break up your workouts by category; cardio and strength training. Try scheduling out your week so you're focusing on a different part of your body each day—arms, legs, abs— and intersperse these with two or three different cardio routines. Having a plan is effective and efficient.

4. Maximize Efficiency

Most people work out in "sets;" doing two to three rounds of a single exercise, interspersed with periods of rest before moving on to a different exercise. Doing a non-stop circuit of one exercise and then moving on to another is far more efficient, allowing muscle groups to rest without lowering the cardiovascular effect by allowing your heart rate to drop. It burns more calories and saves time.

You can even increase the efficiency of your cardio workout. Adding some hills or speed intervals to your running or cycling workout increases your effort and fat-burning, boosts your muscle strength, and burns more calories. If time is a factor in your workout plan, this strategy can help you meet your goals while taking less time out of your busy day.

6

Best Ways to Achieve Weight Loss While Traveling

When you're constantly on the move, traveling for work and pleasure, you may worry that your New Year's weight loss goals will go out the window amid the hustle of hopping planes and changing destinations. Weight loss while traveling is possible, though, if you know the obstacles and plan ahead. Here are some ideas to help you lose weight on the go:

Work Out in Your Room

You'd be amazed to find how many workout routines can be done in the narrow space of a hotel room. You could do jumping jacks and an aerobics workout, stretch, and do a body-weight strength routine. Exercises such as squats, push-ups, chair dips, leg raises and crunches don't require any equipment, but still give you a fulfilling workout to achieve your weight loss goals. You don't have to rely on your own imagination, either—there are a ton of workout apps out there for your mobile device, and many of them allow you to download routines for offline use, so you can even access them without an internet connection.

Walk

Walking is the easiest, most travel-friendly workout there is. Even if you're on business, you'll probably get a little time for some sightseeing. There's no better way to explore a new locale than on foot, and it'll save you plenty in cab fare! Low-impact and excellent for weight loss, it's a perfect way to experience the local atmosphere while burning a ton of calories.

If you're on vacation, book a hotel a little way from the city's center. Not only will you save money, you'll start each day with a built-in workout, and you might even discover some hidden gems while exploring off the beaten path.

Fitness Centers

If your budget allows, choose a hotel with a *good* fitness center. Emphasis on *good*—some hotels will offer you a dingy basement room, with a few hand weights stacked in the corner and a treadmill from the nineties, and call it a gym. Definitely not the sort of atmosphere that inspires an energetic workout! Check out reviews of the fitness center on the booking website, and look for pictures. If your hotel doesn't offer a gym, it might offer complimentary passes or deep discounts for a swanky neighborhood fitness center. Don't be afraid to ask!

Drinking Water

Drinking water is one of those essentials that gets forgotten quickly in the pressure and rush of travel. New places can be overwhelming, and when your routine is disturbed it's easy to forget even the most basic building blocks of your weight loss plan. When you don't drink enough, though, your metabolism gets sluggish, and even if you're keeping up with your diet and exercise, it can be hard to make progress. Try setting an hourly reminder on your phone or watch, and consider bringing one or two reusable bottles you can easily fill from a water fountain, instead of having to walk to the snack bar at the opposite end of the airport. Just remember to make sure your reusable bottle is empty before you go through security, unless you want it confiscated.

Eating Healthy Away From Home

Under stress, hundreds of miles from home, and confronting temptations and unfamiliar foods, it's difficult to maintain healthy eating habits. That doesn't mean you have to subsist on lettuce leaves. Sample the local cuisine and have fun; just make sure the majority of your meals are healthy. A calorie counting app can help you stay on track; they have vast databases of foods with nutritional values built-in.

Avoiding junk calories is key. Instead of grabbing a bag of chips or a candy bar from a bodega, stop at a grocery store and pick up a healthy snack, like a few pieces of fruit or nuts. Lots of restaurants offer health-conscious meal choices, too, and many have websites with nutritional information on their offerings. Take a few minutes before you leave for dinner and choose your meal ahead of time; it can save you hundreds of calories.

With a little preparation and planning, there's no reason why you can't stay on track with your weight loss goals while traveling.

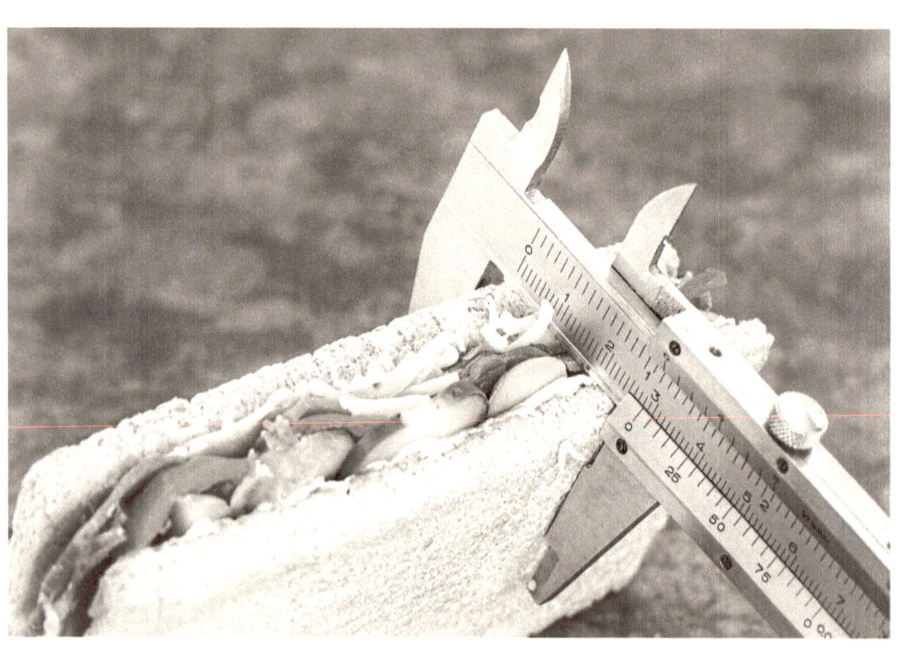

7

An Effective Post-Workout Weight Loss Meal Plan

Post-workout nutrition is an essential part of your weight loss plan. If you don't refuel your body adequately after exercise, your body will go into starvation mode, slowing your metabolism and sabotaging your goals. Conversely, if you don't give your body the right fuel, you'll undo all that hard work you just put into burning calories. It's a fine line, to be sure, but there are plenty of healthy options for a post-workout snack or meal, some of which we've listed below.

When and What to Eat

Most experts agree the best time to eat is thirty to sixty minutes after your workout, when your body is at peak efficiency, supplying protein to your fatigued muscles and replenishing glucose levels. Your best bet is a combination of protein and complex carbohydrates, rich in fiber and low in calories.

Banana Smoothie

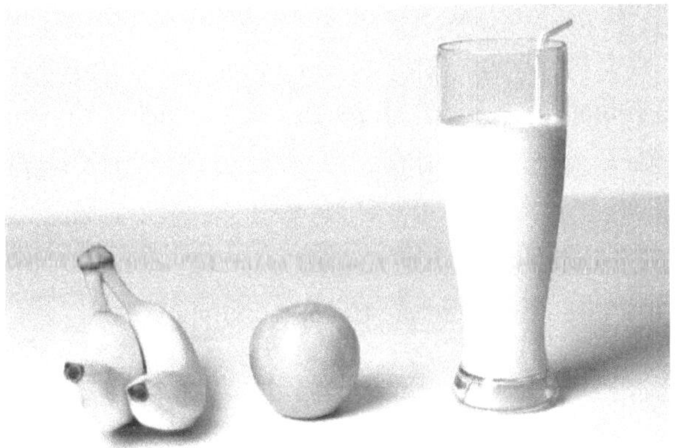

There's no need for added sugar when you blend equal portions of naturally sweet bananas, low-fat milk, and yogurt into a delicious smoothie. You can even add nuts, dried fruit, flaxseed for fiber, or powdered peanut butter for additional flavor.

Creative Sandwiches

Sandwiches are easy to prepare, and the possibilities are endless. Start with fiber- and nutrient-rich whole wheat bread, and add some low-calorie dressing, low sodium cold cuts, and freshly chopped tomatoes, onion and lettuce. Try grilling the sandwich and adding some boiled egg white for an extra treat. With a mix of protein, carbohydrates and vegetables, a sandwich is a perfectly-balanced post-workout meal.

Salmon

Planning meals in advance helps you stick to your goals and gives you a lot more options for your post-workout meal. Grilled salmon with brown rice and steamed vegetables, with a healthy sauce on the side, is a complete, balanced meal and an excellent addition to your menu. Salmon is a great source of protein and vital omega-3 fatty acids, and the veggies and rice will satisfy you with filling fiber.

Peanut Butter

Peanut butter is high in calories and (healthy) fat, but it's an excellent source of protein. As long as you keep an eye on your portion sizes, it can become a tasty component of your post-workout meal or snack. One tablespoon (and remember, a tablespoon is only about the size of a golf ball!) has about 100 calories, but peanut butter's rich flavor goes far. You can add it to a sandwich, or make a wrap with tortillas or Indian *chapattis*, with veggies, eggs, chicken or fish on the side. It's also excellent smeared on apple slices. Another great option is powdered peanut butter, which is pressed and dehydrated, giving you great peanut butter taste with about a quarter of the calories and a small fraction of the fat. Simply rehydrate with water to your preferred consistency, and enjoy!

With all these options, you can't complain that your post-workout meal is boring! With a little creativity, a weight loss meal plan can be full of satisfying flavor that doesn't leave you wanting more.

8

Best Fat Burning Foods for Women

If you're looking for ways to burn fat, and specifically, belly fat, you probably know that diet is more than half the battle. Nearly all health and nutrition experts agree that making sustainable and healthy changes to your diet is the best option to lose weight and keep it off. Extreme fad diets might deliver on rapid weight loss promises, but you don't want to be right back where you started in six months! Burning belly fat with healthy choices and lifestyle changes raises your odds of losing weight and keeping it off for good.

1. Egg Whites

Protein is vital for fat burning, and egg whites are some of the most inexpensive, readily available protein around. Protein sustains and builds muscle, and more muscle mass means a higher resting metabolism, meaning you'll burn more calories just sitting around! Your body has to work harder to break down protein, too, which means more calories spent in the digestive process. Egg whites are as versatile as they are diet-friendly; you can boil them, or scramble them in olive oil with veggies like capsicum and mushrooms. Add some whole wheat bread and a touch of butter, and you've got a healthy, balanced meal.

2. Oatmeal

Among breakfast cereals, oatmeal wins for fat-burning power. It's an excellent source of fiber and healthy, unrefined carbohydrates, which help keep you full and sustain your energy through the morning. It's also relatively low in calories. They're just as versatile as egg whites; for flavor, try brown sugar, fruit or fruit preserves, nuts, and raisins. Steel-cut oats are far healthier than the pressed instant kind, but most people balk at the long cook time, so here's an easy solution—set them up in your slow cooker overnight, and when you wake up, you'll have a warm, ready-to-eat meal.

A side note for new moms trying to lose those post-baby pounds—oatmeal has been linked to increased breast milk production. Not only will you be able to feed your baby more easily, but producing breast milk is a calorie-burner, too!

3. Seasonal Fruits and Vegetables

Finally, a food you can binge on without guilt! Fruits and vegetables are low in calories and rich in healthy carbohydrates, fiber, vitamins and minerals. That means they keep you full and energized, and keep you from reaching for that candy bar.

Eating seasonally is a great way to not only vary your vary and balance your diet, it's also a sustainable way to support your local farmers. Everyone knows about steamed veggies and salads, but there are lots of ways to enjoy them you may not have thought of. You can spiralize zucchini as a low-carb alternative to pasta, rice cauliflower for a guilt-free risotto, and even bake kale leaves with olive oil and sea salt as a replacement for potato chips.

4. Pulses and Beans

Pulses (lentils, chickpeas, etc.) and beans are some of the best vegetarian sources of protein. If you're looking for new ways to enjoy them, look for Indian and Mexican recipes—they make great use of them. There are lots of low-calorie bean and pulse recipes out there, and they're best enjoyed with local whole-wheat breads. You can also roast chickpeas for a crunchy, healthy snack.

5. Lean Meats

You've probably noticed a trend of lean protein on this list, so of course poultry and fish have a place. Try to avoid processed varieties as much as possible. They both go very well with whole wheat pasta, salads, platters, stews and casseroles. Poultry especially is easy to make ahead for busy moms; just throw a few chicken breasts in the slow cooker with some salsa or diced tomatoes and seasoning. Add a different side each day, and you've got lunch or dinner for the whole week.

This list isn't exhaustive, but it's a great starting point, and a good general guideline to point you in the right direction of filling your plate with complex carbohydrates, lean protein, and fiber. Simple, isn't it?

9

Top Foods That Burn Belly Fat

Everyone knows that exercise and especially diet lead to weight loss. But what about *eating* for weight loss? It's not as far-fetched an idea as it might seem. Many foods actually help burn fat, particularly belly fat. Here's a list to help you get started on your fat-burning goals:

Whole Grains

First of all, whole grains have fewer calories than their processed, refined counterparts, like white bread and rice and refined pasta. Additionally, as a source of complex carbohydrates and dietary fiber, whole grains offer sustained energy release, helping you feel fuller longer, and keeping you from overeating. It's best to start with whole grains at breakfast; they may be complex, but they're still carbs, and starting your day with a serving not only helps hold you over until lunch, but gives you the entire day to burn them off. Try a delicious bowl of oatmeal or whole grain cereal, or a slice of whole wheat bread on the side.

Seasonal Fruit

Eating seasonally is good for the environment, your community, and your health. Research has shown that, especially when it comes to fruit, eating seasonally helps to naturally balance your diet. Fruit contains many essential nutrients, but you'll only get them in the right proportions if you vary your consumption.

All fruit contains fiber, which keeps hunger at bay and fills you up, preventing you from overeating. A bowl of fruit is a great answer to your body's craving for sugar, with a lot fewer calories than a bowl of ice cream or a chocolate bar.

Water

It might seem strange to find water on a list of fat-burning *foods,* but there's good reason to include it on this list. Yes, water has zero calories, but that's not what's won it a place on this list; keeping hydrated is crucial for maintaining your metabolism and energy levels. Even mild dehydration leaves you with precious little energy for exercise. Not only that, dehydration cripples your body's crucial post-workout recovery and slows your metabolism. Considering the busy lives most of us lead, though, it's not surprising that we often forget to drink the 8–10 glasses of water experts recommend for optimal hydration, especially since, by the time you're thirsty, you're already dehydrated. Try this—line up eight pennies on one side of the windowsill in your kitchen. Every time you drink a glass of water, slide a penny to the opposite side. Or, if you're on the move, set an hourly reminder on your watch or mobile device. It's difficult to form a new habit, but after a few weeks, reaching for a glass of water every hour or so will become second-nature.

Lean Meats

Lean meats such as chicken or seafood are a great source of protein. Protein is essential for building lean muscle, boosting your metabolism, and keeping hunger pangs at bay. It's also free of inessential fats and junk calories.

Beans and Legumes

If you're a vegetarian or vegan, beans and legumes are some of the best sources of low-fat protein, particularly if you're trying to lose weight. Even if you're not a vegetarian, they'll add variety and nutrients to your fat-burning diet. Combined with whole grains, beans and legumes offer almost the same amino acid combination as lean meats.

Green Leafy Vegetables

Spinach isn't just for Popeye! Leafy greens are low in calories and rich in fiber, the ideal weight loss combination, and they offer many essential nutrients as well.

Just remember the greener the better—iceberg lettuce's mild flavor makes it a popular salad choice, but it's the vegetable equivalent of white bread where nutrients are concerned. Darker greens have higher concentrations of vitamins, so they pack a one-two punch of fiber and nutrition.

While by no means an exhaustive list of belly fat-burning foods, this should give you an idea of the sort of nutrition you should be focusing on to start losing weight and regaining your health.

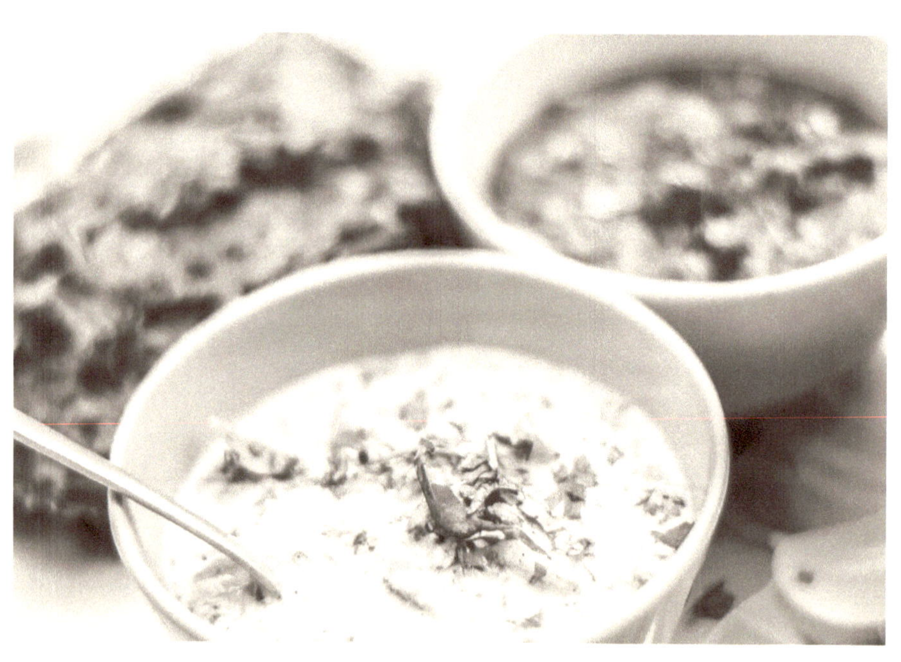

10

An Indian Vegetarian Diet for Weight Loss and Good Health: Does It Work?

India is a paradise for vegetarians. There are hundreds of vegetarian Indian recipes, and it's one of the few cultures where meat and cheese aren't essential components of a main meal. Indian cooking gives you the opportunity to utilize vegetables in ways you might never have imagined. Blended with local herbs and spices and swimming in delectable curries, if cooked properly, these vegetables retain their freshness and distinct flavor. It's no wonder an Indian vegetarian diet works so well for weight loss!

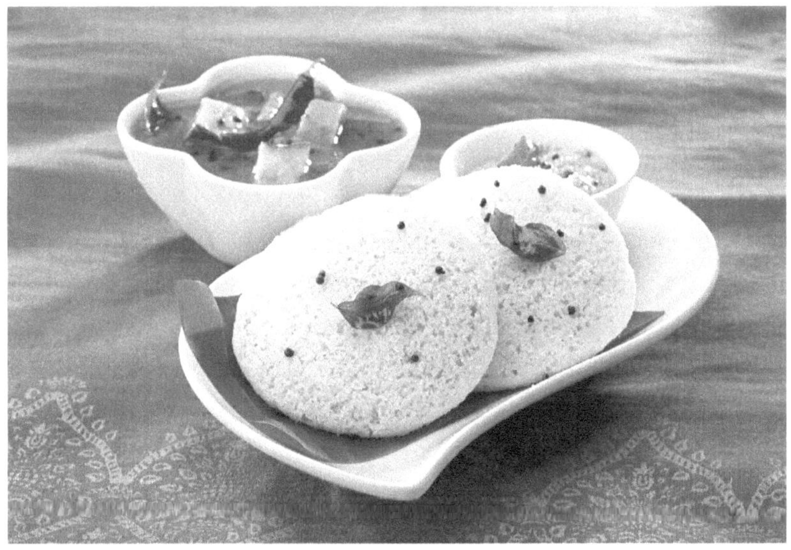

Indian Cooking Works for Weight Loss!

If cooked correctly, Indian meals are at once light, nutritious, and filling. It's the excessive use of clarified butter, or *ghee,* fatty vegetable oils, deep-fried snacks, and high-sugar sweets which are responsible for obesity in India. Fortunately, none of these are essential to Indian cooking.

Substitute *Ghee* With Olive or Vegetable Oil

This is the first step if you're following an Indian vegetarian diet for weight loss. *Ghee* is rich in saturated fat and, if consumed in excess, slows your metabolism and leads to obesity. Olive and other vegetable oils are far healthier, and grocery store aisles are now filled with health-conscious varieties free of saturated fats.

Cooking Methods With Minimal Oil

Cooking methods have a huge impact on how healthy and low-calorie your Indian meal turns out to be. Most Indian recipes begin by sautéing onions, garlic, ginger and various herbs and spices in oil before adding puree or cream. Instead, try blanching onions rather than frying them. Spices can be dry-roasted in a frying pan to bring out their flavor, and non-stick spray can be used instead of a heavy dollop of oil.

Using Milk and Dairy

Most Indians can't imagine preparing a meal without milk or dairy products. Fresh cream, yogurt, milk, pressed cottage cheese (*paneer*) and butter are all staples of an Indian pantry. Fortunately, milk and dairy products are also an essential part of a balanced diet and weight loss plan, as long as you choose a low-fat option. Most commercially available Indian dairy products, including *paneer* and yogurt, are prepared from full-fat milk, but you can make this yourself at home from low-fat milk. It's easier than you think!

Make *Chapatti* Your Staple Bread

Chapatti is cooked whole-wheat flat bread, a staple in many Indian households. It's healthy, low-calorie, and a great source of fiber and complex carbohydrates for energy and fullness. Just use restraint when it comes to adding *ghee* or butter; this simple step will save you a ton of calories. Save more calorie-rich *naan* and *paranthas* breads for special occasions.

Brown Rice Rather Than White

Refined white rice may be more popular and readily obtainable than brown, but brown rice has fewer calories and is more nutritious. Experiment with seasonings, and it'll soon be your new, healthy staple.

No matter your reason for adopting an Indian vegetarian diet, remember to exercise portion control, and you'll see results in no time.

11

Eating Out and Weight Loss: the Restaurant Foods to Avoid at All Costs!

Many people hesitate to start a diet plan because they believe they'll end up stuck at home, eating bland, regimented meals. But eating out and weight loss aren't as incompatible as you might think. Knowledge is power; if you can avoid the top 'restaurant evils,' you can meet your weight loss goals and still have fun!

Sodas

Sodas are the obvious place to start, because they're the first thing you order when you arrive at a restaurant. You probably already know that soda is nothing more than empty calories and deadly chemicals. Most people drink soda out of habit or availability, not taste—a few weeks off them, and you'll realize they didn't taste all that great in the first place. Cutting soda will easily reduce your calories by 200–350 per meal. There are plenty of healthier options on the menu, such as hot or unsweetened iced tea, or, of course, water.

Juices

When you think of healthy beverages, juice probably comes to mind. Sadly, most juices are processed and sweetened, loaded with empty sugar calories, and hardly better than soda. While juices contain the water and sugar from fruit, the juicing process removes most of the fiber, vitamins and minerals, removing the components which make fruit such a healthy diet choice and turning it into an unsatisfying glass of empty calories. Starting your meal with a fresh fruit salad is a far healthier option.

Fried Foods

Giving into your craving for a burger doesn't have to mean wrecking your diet. Most of the time it's not the burger sabotaging your goals, it's the French fries or chips on the side. Deep-fried foods are calorie bombs, and most of those calories come from unhealthy fats. Try having your burger with a fresh side salad or plate of steamed veggies instead. Even fast-food restaurants now offer salads as a healthy alternative to fries or onion rings. Add a mildly-sweetened iced tea instead of soda, and you've just saved yourself up to 900 calories.

Refined Foods

Whether you're eating out or dining in, processed, refined foods should be high on your 'avoid' list. Stay away from large portions of rice and pasta, ignore the loaf of white bread and butter meant to hold you over until the meal arrives (or ask the server to take it away, if you can't trust yourself!), and whenever possible, opt for whole-wheat bread, pasta or brown rice with your meal. Even if it's not on the menu, most restaurants are happy to make substitutions, so don't be afraid to ask.

Portion Control

This might just be the worst enemy of a 'dieting while dining out' plan. Restaurant portions are *huge*. Put into perspective, a serving of meat or protein should be around the size of a deck of cards; your carbohydrate serving about the size of your closed fist. Now compare these to your last meal out, and you'll quickly see the problem. There's an easy solution, though—ask your server to bring a to-go box with your meal. Before you start eating, put half of everything on your plate into the box. Not only are you now eating an appropriate portion, but you have lunch for tomorrow, too!

If you eat out ten times a month, you could lose two or three pounds easily by following these tips. A bit of restraint and knowledge is all you need to reach your weight loss goals while having fun, too!

12

Desk Exercises to Lose Weight Fast

Trying to balance work, family, and a social life is hard enough without trying to find time to exercise, which is why many people write it off as a lost cause. But you don't need to work out for two hours a day to see results. What really matters is the cumulative value of exercise. Provided you're following a healthy diet plan, even fifteen minutes of exercise a day will lead to weight loss. You might not see the same dramatic results as you would from hitting the gym five days a week, but a few small changes can still give you results. These easy but effective desk exercises are a great way to start losing a few extra pounds.

Stretching

Stretching is extremely important to combat stiffness and injuries and improve your muscles' range of motion. Stiff muscles can quickly become injuries, which can seriously derail your exercise and weight loss program. You don't need a full yoga routine to loosen up, though; these stretches can be done without even leaving your desk.

Touch the floor – Remain seated in your chair and plant your feet in a wide, stable position. Raise your arms straight above your head as high as you can, palms facing each other. Now, keeping your torso straight and stretched, hinge forward from the hips and touch the floor between your feet, breathing deeply and steadily. For this exercise, remain seated in your chair and plant your feet in a wide and stable position. Hold the stretch for two to five seconds, and then slowly return to sitting. Repeat five times.

Stretch your sides — Raise your arms, interlock your fingers and push your palms up toward the ceiling. Bend slightly to one side, hold for two to five seconds, return to center, and repeat on the other side. Do this five times on each side.

Muscle Toning

Now that your body is stretched and ready for action, you can try some cardio and muscle-toning exercises while at your desk.

Chair Dips — This is a great exercise for your upper body, particularly for those often-neglected triceps. Make sure your chair is stable, and then grip the sides of the seat and slide forward off the chair, keeping your knees bent as though still seated. Bend your elbows and lower your body a few inches. Hold for a moment, and then push back up into your floating seated position. Repeat this exercise eight to ten times.

Chair Squats — Chair squats are some of the easiest and most challenging exercises you can do for your core muscles and lower body. Stand up in front of your chair, feet shoulder-width apart. Now, lower your body until you feel your backside just touch the chair. Hold for two to five seconds, and then return to standing without using the chair or desk for support. Repeat eight to ten times.

Cardiovascular Exercises

Even if you do cardio for sixty seconds at a time, it'll still burn calories and help you get slim. All you need is an empty room or a bit of space near your desk for a minute of jumping jacks or vigorous running in place. You can also try a few rounds of stair climbing or a brisk walk around your office during lunch hour.

If you're willing to invest a few dollars, you can take 'desk fitness' even further. You can buy an under-desk elliptical or bicycle to keep your legs moving while you work. This could even improve your work performance; studies done on schoolchildren have shown that putting them on a stationary bicycle with a desk in class improved their test scores and overall concentration. Also, swapping out your desk chair for an exercise ball will keep your core muscles engaged and improve your posture while you sit at your desk. You can get a base for the ball, too, so it doesn't roll away every time you get up. Companies are becoming more and more aware of the effects of constant sitting on their employees' health, and they know that healthy employees are more productive and miss less work, so many are quite receptive to workers taking these initiatives to improve their health.

If you stay consistent with these simple exercises, you'll be feeling stronger and more energetic in no time, all while shedding excess calories.

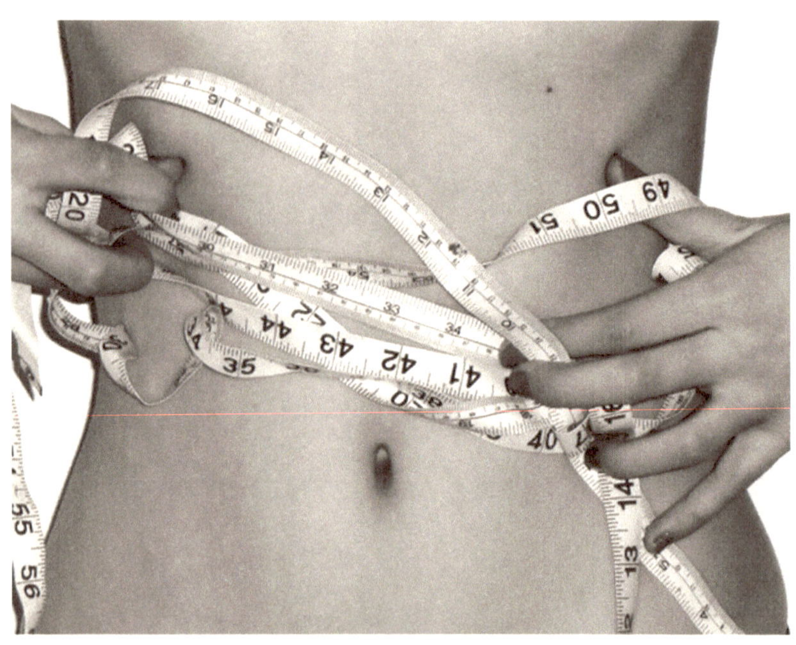

13

5 Essential Tips to Lose Belly Fat Fast

The internet is full of "expert" articles telling us a healthy diet and exercise are the best ways to lose belly fat. They're certainly not wrong, but such generalized tips can hardly work miracles for the average person, already struggling to keep up with the challenges of a hectic home and work life. What you really need is a specific plan of action, to help you begin when you have no idea where to start. Below are some effective tips to lose belly fat with minimum disruption to your life.

Blend Exercise Into Your Life

Even if you can't find the time to exercise right now, you don't have to put off your weight loss goals. Start getting your body accustomed to exercise by using the stairs instead of the elevator, taking a brisk walk to run your errands instead of driving or taking the bus, or parking your car a block away from work. Not only will you strengthen your muscles, but you'll burn extra calories with hardly any effect on your normal day. Don't be surprised if you start losing weight already!

Make It Short and Intense

If your schedule allows time for exercise, maximize the benefit of that time with interval training. Rather than jogging at one pace for thirty minutes, intersperse your jog with two or three evenly-timed, fast-paced intervals. For instance, after warming up, you could do a thirty-second sprint, followed by a sixty-second jog. Continue these sets for as long as you have energy in the tank. Interval training has been proven not only to burn more calories during exercise, but raise your metabolic rate to continue burning higher levels of calories for up to sixty minutes after your workout.

Control Stress and Get Enough Sleep

If you don't get enough sleep, your metabolism will slow, and you won't have the energy to exercise, seriously cutting down on the number of calories you'll burn. Lack of sleep is also linked to elevated levels of the stress hormone cortisol, which causes your body to store excess levels of belly fat.

When you're stressed, you make poor decisions, and that applies to food as much as anything else. Stressed-out people are more likely to binge on comfort food, which can undo weeks of hard work. If you're trying to focus on exercise and diet, ignoring your sleep and stress levels means you're fighting a losing battle.

Snack Healthy

We can all manage reasonably healthy meals with a bit of effort, but what seems to be most people's downfall is snacks. Rather than a burger, chips, or sugary, packaged food, keep some fruit and a handful of raisins and nuts to fight those afternoon hunger pangs, or some peanut butter with whole-wheat crackers or apple slices. Healthy snacking can save you up to 500 calories a day, and that adds up to 4 ½ pounds a month!

14

Vital Diet Tips to Burn Fat in the Face and Achieve Younger Skin

You can hide a muffin top under a loose sweater and high-waisted jeans, but you can't disguise chubby cheeks and a double chin. Excess facial fat can add years to your appearance, but we have some tips to help melt it away and make you look younger in a matter of weeks.

Why Your Face Looks Puffy and Fat

A puffy face isn't just the result of fat. Saggy, loose skin means your skin has lost elasticity; premature aging, in other words, brought on by toxins in your body and hormone imbalances. With the right diet, you can brighten and firm your skin as well as losing facial weight.

Omit Processed Foods

Processed, packaged foods are full of salt, chemicals, and toxic additives, which are largely responsible for hormonal imbalances and symptoms of premature aging. Natural, raw and unprocessed foods, on the other hand, are rich in minerals and antioxidants which flush out your system and prevent toxin buildups.

Include Fruits and Vegetables

This is one reason health and nutrition experts harp constantly to add more fruits and vegetables to your diet. There is no diet richer in vitamins and minerals than one with a balanced variety of seasonal fruits and vegetables.

Also, fruits and vegetables are rich in fiber, low in calories, and have a high water content, which help you lose facial fat fast. The fiber keeps you full, the low calorie density ensures you don't overeat, and the water content helps flush salts and toxins from your tissues. The more water weight and actual fat you burn through diet and exercise, the slimmer your face will become.

Drink Water

As we just mentioned, water flushes toxins from your body and keeps you replenished and hydrated. Getting rid of those toxins is the only way to young, firm, glowing skin, and it's impossible to do if you're not drinking enough water. Unless your skin looks tight and healthy, all your efforts to lose facial fat will be for nothing.

Your body might also interpret thirst as hunger while dehydrated, leading to consumption of unnecessary calories. A dehydrated body is has a sluggish metabolism, too, meaning it certainly won't be able to burn off those extra calories you consume. So, to lose facial fat fast, make sure you drink 7–9 tall glasses of water every day.

Don't Ignore Proteins

Finally, if you're looking to lose facial fat, lean proteins should be a staple of your diet. Proteins help maintain and build muscle in your body, especially if you help them by exercising, and muscle speeds up metabolism, helping you burn through fat reserves faster. The best lean sources of protein are soy, lentils, beans and legumes, eggs, dairy, chicken and fish.

15

The Role of Genetics in Weight Loss and Fat Burning

An important aspect of losing weight fast is identifying your body type. There are three different body types: ectomorphs, endomorphs, and mesomorphs. All three have different strengths, weaknesses, and needs, and by identifying these, you can lose weight faster and reshape your body. Here, we'll help you identify your body type, and give you the best strategies for weight loss without frustration.

Ectomorphs

Ectomorphs are naturally lean, with a narrow bone structure and long limbs. It's quite rare for ectomorphs to put on weight, since they have a rapid metabolism and generally struggle to put on weight, or even muscle. The good news is that, if an ectomorph does gain weight, it'll come off quickly and easily.

An ectomorph's naturally fast metabolism works to their advantage. All he or she needs to do in order to lose weight fast is to cut junk food, sugary sweets, and alcohol from their diet, and incorporate three or four thirty-minute cardio sessions into their weekly routine. Ectomorphs should concentrate on exercises that build lean muscle, like dance or yoga. Even a busy ectomorph with no time for exercise will reap productive results simply by incorporating more activity, such as taking the stairs or walking or biking to work, into their daily routine.

Often, however, ectomorphs are more concerned with gaining weight, especially muscle. If that's the case for you, cut down on cardio (no more than one or two sessions per week) and instead focus on short, intense bursts of weight lifting with heavy weights. You'll need to feed those growing muscles with a protein-rich diet, and make sure you consume more calories than you burn in a day. You'll be eating a lot, but make sure to focus on the quality of the food you eat.

Endomorphs

Endomorphs are characterized by rounded, curvy bodies, a heavier bone structure, and a higher percentage of body fat. They have a hard time losing weight, and a hard time keeping it off. They're often plagued by fatigue as well, which can derail their exercise plans. Since this is the body type most likely to become overweight, if you're reading this book, you're most likely an endomorph.

Don't be discouraged by all the negatives, though. Endomorphs also build muscle relatively easily, and once they're in shape, women usually have a beautiful, full-hipped hourglass figure, while men will develop a broad-shouldered, thick-muscled physique. The key is not only to lose weight, but to develop a lifelong healthy eating and exercise plan to keep the weight off for good, which of course has many benefits other than outward appearance. Lean protein will work for you, too, but make sure your carbohydrates are complex and as unrefined as possible. Stick to oatmeal and whole grain breads. And be prepared to eat a *ton* of fruits and vegetables. You'll need to count every calorie, so invest in a meal diary or download a calorie-tracker app.

In terms of exercise, endomorphs should focus on high-intensity cardio, particularly interval training, like HIIT, tabata, or even martial arts. You'll need to be consistent if you want to see results, though, so consider enrolling in classes at a gym near you, so you're committed to a time and place. Stay hydrated and get plenty of sleep, too, to combat that endomorphic fatigue.

Mesomorphs

The most balanced body type is a mesomorph. Without a doubt, they're the winners of the body-type lottery. They have a natural propensity toward a strong, muscular body and athletic build, with a perfect frame and good posture. Female mesomorphs generally have a natural hourglass figure and plenty of lean muscle.

Their metabolisms are fast, and their muscles develop easily. That doesn't mean they don't need to look after their health, though—no body type can stand up to sustained abuse and neglect.

Mesomorphs will lose weight quickly, as long as they stay disciplined with a healthy diet and a balanced exercise regime. Their meal plan and dietary needs are similar to an ectomorph's, only they'll need to watch their calories more closely, and add more cardio to their fitness plan.

Bear in mind that not all people fit neatly into one of these three categories. Most people are a mixture of two types, with primary characteristics from one and secondary characteristics from another. A good trainer and nutritionist should be able to help you figure out your body type. Knowledge is power, and soon you'll be on your way to the physique you've always dreamed of.

16

Looking for Fast Weight Loss – Lose Weight Permanently with Anaerobic Exercise

Most people don't just want to lose weight fast, they want to keep it off permanently, so establishing a lifelong exercise plan is crucial. For many people, though, choosing an exercise plan which gives them lasting weight loss results might not be as simple as just choosing one off a list. Many people can jog for 2–3 hours a week without making any tangible progress with their weight loss goals. It might be because they're not doing anaerobic exercise. According to several studies, people who incorporate anaerobic exercise into their routines have a far better chance of achieving their weight loss goals.

What Is Anaerobic Exercise?

During anaerobic exercise, the body's muscles are supplied with very little oxygen. Muscle training with medium-to-heavy weights, sprinting, and cycling or swimming at maximum speed are all examples of anaerobic exercises, as you can only sustain this degree of effort for a few minutes. Aerobic exercises, however, such as steady jogs and cycling, or swimming, can be sustained for several minutes or even hours, because the muscles are supplied with sufficient oxygen.

Why Anaerobic Exercise Helps You Lose Weight Fast

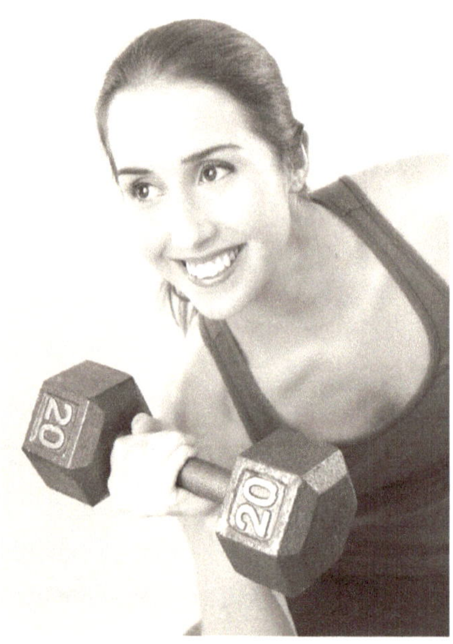

Aerobic exercise burns calories from carbohydrates first. Only when they've been depleted will they start to burn fat. Your body will demand replenishment after your workout, though, and if you replace all the calories you just burned, it was a wasted effort. With anaerobic exercise, though, your muscles only feel the strain for a few minutes, and then the body immediately gets to work repairing and growing them. It's hard work, and your body needs a lot of calories to make it happen, calories it'll use up both during and *after* your workout. So, while you're fast asleep at night, your body is actually burning calories and losing weight. It's no wonder that people who incorporate anaerobic exercise into their regime usually lose weight permanently.

Any expert will tell you that no aerobic exercise will help you burn calories while you're at rest. But anaerobic exercise does, both in the short and the long term. Once your muscles are well-developed, your basic metabolic rate (the rate at which you burn calories while doing nothing) will rise, due to the effort of feeding and supporting those muscles. The bigger the muscles, the bigger the burn!

Anaerobic is for Everyone

The best part is that you don't need to bench press 200 pounds, or spend hours on the track doing 200 meter sprints to get your anaerobic exercise. Even moderate weight lifting counts as anaerobic exercise. If you do two to three sets of an exercise as part of a circuit, with ten to twelve reps in each set, that's more than enough to start seeing the benefits of anaerobic exercise. And don't worry, ladies—you're not going to end up with massive, bulky muscles. Your body simply doesn't produce enough testosterone to turn you into a beefcake. What you will achieve is a more toned and shapely body, and faster weight loss.

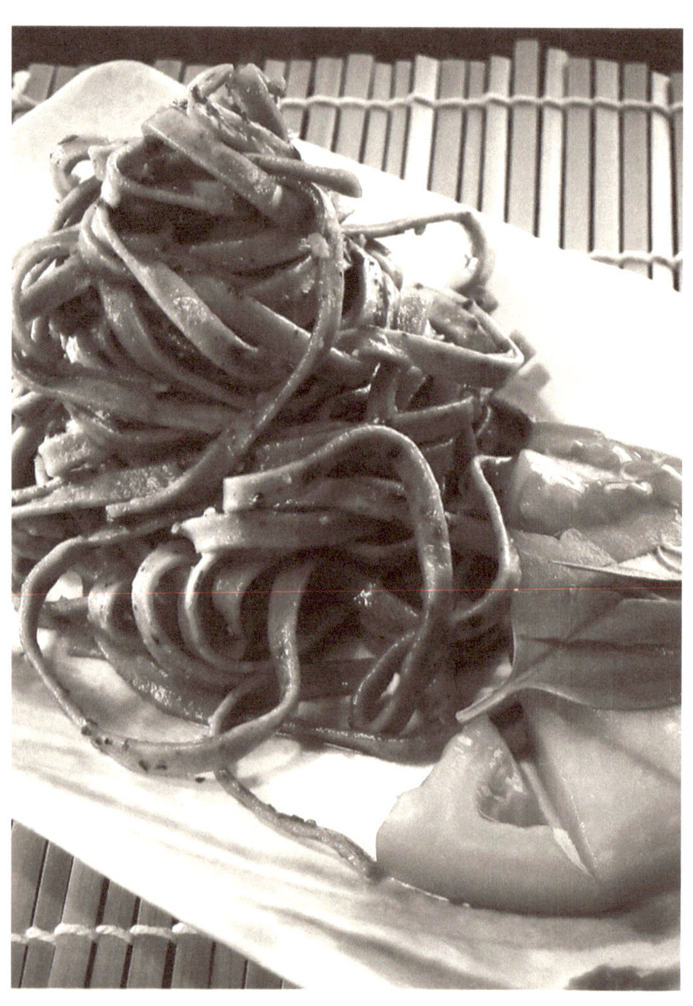

17

6 Tips on a Practical Diet for Weight Loss in Women Over 40

If you're over forty, you might think your chances for losing weight are as slim as you'd like to be. But if you're aware of the challenges, and the proven techniques to overcome them, you have no reason to feel disheartened. This is your opportunity to regain your health and strength for all the years that lie ahead.

The Challenges

First, you need to accept that weight loss won't be as easy as it would be for someone in their twenties. You'll need to put in a more committed effort, since you're fighting pre-menopausal hormone imbalances and declining muscle mass, both of which slow your metabolism. It's extremely important to control your calorie consumption, and make healthy, sustainable changes to your diet.

1. Foods to Avoid

Your body is no longer as efficient as it was in processing carbohydrate-rich or fatty foods. Slow down on fried, processed foods and meals high in sugar. Alcohol is another especially stealthy diet downfall, so cut down on cocktails, wine and beer.

2. The Best Foods for Weight Loss

As with any diet, you need to incorporate lots of lean protein and fiber-rich foods to lose weight successfully in your forties. Lean meats, legumes and beans, egg whites, skim milk and other low-fat dairy products, soy and nuts are all healthy choices which can be dressed up in a number of ways to satisfy any palate. Fruits, vegetables, and whole grain cereals and bread are necessary, too, for that essential fiber to fill you up without filling up on calories.

3. Benefits of Protein

Protein revives your declining muscle mass and, by proxy, your metabolism. Protein-rich foods are filling, and take longer to break down during digestion, which means they'll satisfy for hours after your meal, preventing the urge to reach for a snack. The additional work your body puts into digestion also means more resting calories burned.

4. Fiber Rich Foods

In addition to keeping you full with their abundant fiber, whole grains, fruits, and vegetables are packed with vital nutrients which are crucial for hormone balance and overall good health. And just like a well-tuned car engine, a healthy body will operate at maximum efficiency.

5. Calcium

If you're not a fan of dairy, you need to know that you're missing out on a major calcium source which, as you age, is crucial to maintaining bone density. Calcium is also abundant in spinach and other leafy green vegetables, beans, legumes, almonds, oranges and peas. Bone health is especially important now, as you're most likely beginning to exercise to speed your weight-loss goals. The very definition of exercise is putting your body under stress, so your body needs a strong support system.

6. The Myth Busted

You might have to put some work into it, but there is no irresolvable conflict between 'healthy' and 'tasty.' It's a myth, and a damaging one, which has stopped many women's weight-loss goals in their tracks before they even began. There are lots of exciting flavors and hundreds, maybe even thousands of healthy, tasty recipes out there. Whole wheat pancakes, scrambled eggs in olive oil with capsicum and mushroom, oatmeal with chopped fruits and nuts, low-calorie muesli and fruit salad are all delicious, healthy options for breakfast. As for the rest of the day, there are a range of easy-to-prepare meals, platters, and salads. You can have a lot of fun with your food while still working toward your weight loss goals.

18

Losing Weight Can Improve Your Sex Drive and Strengthen Your Relationship

The list of health benefits of losing weight are endless, and here's one more—if low sex drive is one of your problems, losing weight might solve it. Many sexual health experts agree that losing weight is a sure way to improve your sex drive and performance.

The Physical Connection Between Excess Weight and Low Libido

Excess weight often causes high cholesterol and insulin resistance. One of the side effects of these conditions is poor circulation; they shut down the blood vessels leading to the penis and the clitoris. Without adequate blood flow, an affected individual will experience lack of sensation and possibly impotence. Weight loss, achieved with healthy diet and regular exercise, proper blood flow is restored, correcting these conditions.

Healthy Diet and Sex Drive

Weight loss boosts your libido dramatically, but even if you haven't started to lose weight yet, a healthier diet will work wonders for your performance in the bedroom. With lower cholesterol and increased insulin sensitivity, that blood flow is already returning to the sexual organs, and an improvement in your body's fuel means you'll have more energy and stamina.

Exercise and Sex Drive

Exercise has a direct effect on improving sex drive, since it controls stress, improves lean muscle mass, and increases energy. All of these improve your performance between the sheets!

The Psychological Connection Between Weight Loss and Sex

When talking about the effect of weight loss on libido, it's impossible to ignore the psychological aspects. In modern culture, where the media and peers constantly emphasize and campaign for a lean figure, overweight people are very conscious about their appearance. This is especially true for women. After all, when you're obsessing about how your thighs or stomach look, you can't let go and enjoy the moment, and sex is all about enjoying the moment. While on your weight loss journey, it's also important to start thinking more positively about yourself, and adopt a deeper view of your own sensuality. Rediscovering your sex drive has as much to do with your mind as it does with your body.

Sex experts have also found that, when people begin to take responsibility for their own health, they begin to feel better and more confident about themselves in general. This reduces their stress levels, and increases their desire for sex. Essentially, taking steps to lose weight is an expression of your determination to be in control of your life and destiny. This sort of mindset is important when it comes to sex, as well.

Losing weight can improve your sex drive and strengthen your relationship, but it's important to remember that, just because you're overweight, that doesn't mean that you are or should be incapable of enjoying sex or performing in bed. According to a study in the US, 70% of overweight people continue to report a healthy sex life. There are plenty of reasons to lose weight; if sex isn't already one of them, there's no reason to create problems where they don't exist!

19

Cycling as a Successful Way to Lose Weight Fast

When people realize they're overweight, they tend to push the panic button and make all sorts of drastic lifestyle changes to lose weight fast. But these panic-driven decisions are neither healthy nor sustainable, and will only lead to failure. When it comes to weight loss success, it's the realistic, long-term changes that count. Instead of trying for six-week miracles, make a small change and measure the effect it'll have over the next six months to a year. Biking can be one of those small changes which yield great results over time!

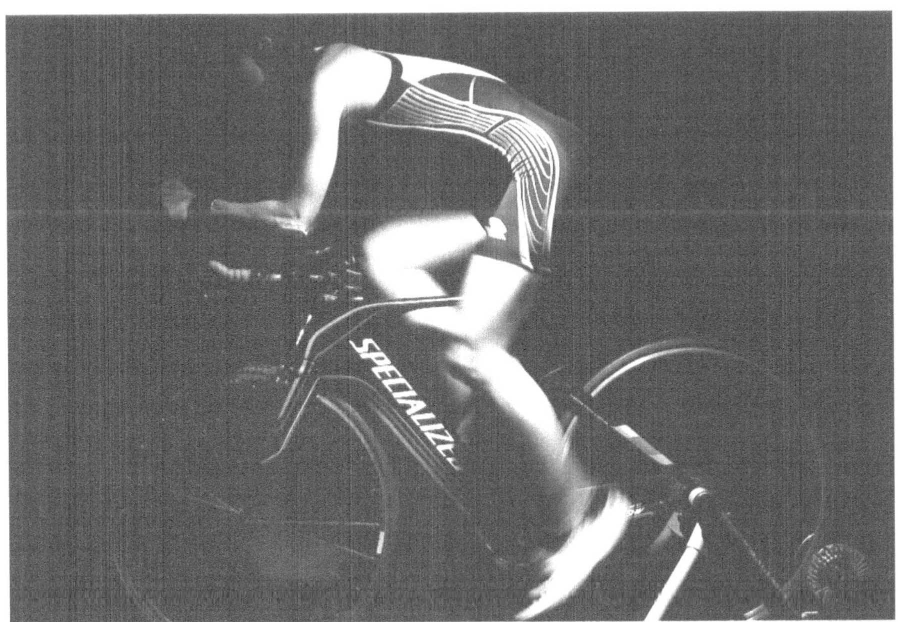

The Mathematics of Cycling and Weight Loss

One pound of body weight equals 3500 calories. So, if you burn 3500 more calories than you consume in the space of a month, you'll lose one pound. Biking at a leisurely pace burns about 450 calories per hour. So, if your diet is healthy and wholesome, and if you do an hour of cycling four times a week, you'll lose four pounds in a month. It may not sound like much, but four pounds a month is 24 pounds in six months, and 48 in one year! That's nearly fifty pounds due to a sustainable, enjoyable change in your lifestyle.

The Advantages

Cycling will also improve your overall muscle tone and mass, if you supplement it with the right diet. More muscle means more calories burned, even while at rest. So, even while sitting on your couch or at your desk at work the day after your ride, your body is burning more calories than it normally would. So, not only does cycling burn more calories while you're doing it, but it gives your metabolism an overall boost.

Some Biking Ideas

Not only is biking a great weight loss idea, it's fun, and easy to incorporate into your life. Instead of driving or using public transportation, why not bicycle to work? You can use your bike to run errands, too, and explore new places with family and friends. Weekend rides are a great opportunity to meet new people and go on excursions and picnics. The great advantage of cycling is that it fits neatly into your routine, without having to designate separate time for exercise.

Higher Intensity Training

As you get used to bicycling, so does your body. It's now adapted to the intensity of your workout, and expending less energy on your usual bicycle commute to work, which means fewer calories burned. Now, try increasing the intensity of your cycling workout by incorporating fast-paced intervals, or sprints, into your ride. This will boost both your overall fitness and your metabolism. Plan a faster burst between two landmarks to start, such as traffic junctions or pillars, and gradually increase the number of intervals as you notice yourself getting less winded after each.

Don't let yourself sink into a fixed and rigid workout routine. Rediscover the kid in you, be adventurous on your bicycle, and you'll find a fun, successful way to lose weight fast.

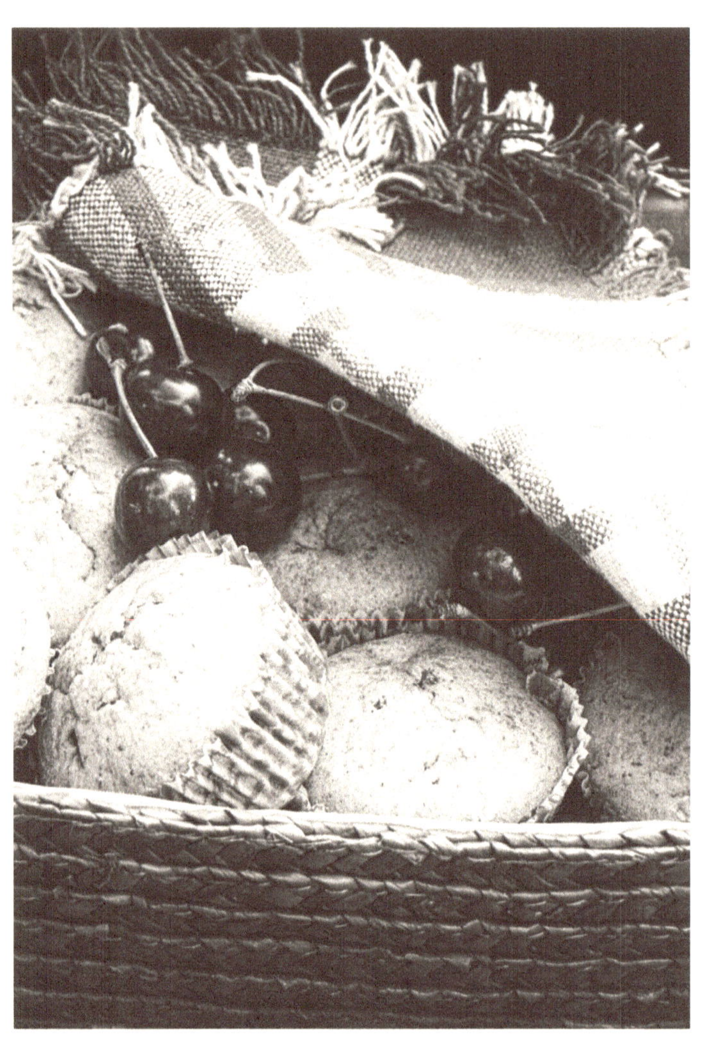

20

5 Tips for Eating Out Without Compromising Your Weight Loss Efforts

After a lot of weight loss diet fads have come and gone over the years, most nutritionists have realized that the most sustainable long-term solution for a healthy and lean body is a simple, balanced diet. However, maintaining such a diet means exercising discipline and portion control, especially with regards to eating out without compromising your weight loss efforts.

The Danger of Malls and Movie Theaters

A shopping trip to the mall is almost invariably followed by a visit to the food court, and a trip to the movies just isn't complete without a soda and popcorn. A large tub of popcorn and soda, though, or a steak meal with fries, can cost you 1000–1200 calories. Even if you just stop for a snack, cinnamon rolls, sandwiches, shakes, and even some flavored coffees measure in at over 500 calories each. A single fun outing can seriously disrupt your weight loss efforts, without you even realizing it.

Carry Healthy Snacks

Start making it a habit to put a few healthy snacks in your purse or pocket, like an apple or a handful of nuts. High-fiber snacks like these will fight hunger pangs, and make it easier to resist temptation. Remember to stay hydrated, too—it's easy to forget to drink enough in an air-conditioned mall, but your body may confuse thirst for hunger and convince you to overeat.

Kids' Meals are Your Best Bet

Without a measuring cup or scale, it's very difficult to measure portion sizes on the go. Here's a simple hack—order a small or kids' meal instead of a regular or large. Restaurant portion sizes have increased over the years, and what was once considered a fair helping for adults is now labeled kids' size. No wonder Americans are getting fatter!

Value Meal Deals Are a Trap!

By restricting yourself to small burgers, sandwiches, popcorn or meals, you'll be able to satisfy your taste buds and still exercise portion control. Whatever you do, don't fall for the temptation of value meal combos offering savings on sodas or fries. It might save you money, but you'll pay in added sugar, fat, and calories. And of course, it should go without saying to steer clear of the buffet. Don't resist temptation, *avoid* it.

Weight Loss while Eating Out at Restaurants

With a growing number of health-conscious customers, many restaurants now offer meals with calorie counts in mind, so don't hesitate to ask your server for the lightest and most nutritious choices.

Dinner entrees are larger than lunch servings, and most restaurants are happy to accommodate requests for lunch portions at any time of day. Another effective strategy is to ask your server to pack half your meal for takeout. Eat slowly and sip water between mouthfuls, and you'll soon realize half of a hefty restaurant portion is more than enough. Portion control isn't about starving yourself; it's about not eating more than your body requires.

21

Your Weight Loss Solution – Exercise Portion Control for Weight Loss!

Following a specialized weight loss meal plan isn't always a practical or effective weight loss solution. Prepping special meals takes time, effort and even money most people can't afford. In any case, most nutritionists will tell you that, if you keep your diet wholesome and balanced, that should be good enough to control your calorie intake, provided you keep your portions in check. With a bit of focus, discipline, and knowledge, it's easy to exercise portion control during meals.

Eat Consistently

Considering how busy most of us are, it's easy to ignore our body's needs and skip meals. This is counterproductive, though; your hunger will return with a vengeance at night, and you'll likely end up overeating at the worst possible time of the day, affecting your sleep, your metabolism, and your weight loss efforts. Speaking of timing, portion control for weight loss is most essential for dinner; it should be your lightest meal of the day, and that will only be feasible when you've fueled your body consistently throughout the day.

The Benefit of Healthy Snacks

Meals aren't the only place to apply consistent eating. Having healthy, low-calorie snacks throughout the day will keep you satisfied without overloading you with calories, and help you control your meal portions. Fruit, a handful of nuts, whole-grain crackers and a light sandwich on whole-wheat bread all make good snacks to keep you feeling satisfied and in control.

Drink Water Frequently

As we've already mentioned, the body often interprets thirst as hunger, so staying hydrated keeps your body from getting confused. Also, a full glass of water before every meal fills your stomach and slows digestion, so you'll reach satiety sooner and feel full longer.

Portion Control When You Are Distracted

Scheduling meals during quiet time when you won't be interrupted is best, because it allows you to concentrate on your food and lets your brain sync up to your stomach. Self-awareness lets you pick up on fullness cues faster, instead of mindlessly shoveling more mouthfuls into your already full stomach. If you're going to be unavoidably distracted during your meal, make sure to carefully measure your portion beforehand, instead of bringing the whole bag of chips into the living room.

Eating Slowly

A related tip is eating slowly. It can take your brain fifteen-twenty minutes to get your stomach's signal that it's full. When you eat slowly, you allow your body time to digest and register fullness. It's very difficult to exercise portion control if you eat rapidly, since before you know it, you'll have eaten more than your body needs.

If, at the end of a meal, you still feel hungry, drink a glass of water and wait ten minutes before going for seconds. Most of the time, you'll realize you didn't need that second helping after all.

If you're mindful of your body's signals and your portion sizes, you can likely save yourself 300–400 calories a day—considering that amount can make you put on three pounds a month, that's not an insignificant number!

22

Lose Weight Without Going on a Diet? – Follow These 3 Food Tips

The nourishment you provide your body produces direct consequences, whether that's a lean, strong body or rolls of fat. Consistently denying yourself food or severely limiting your calories can lead to weakness, fatigue, illness, and a slower metabolism, which will come back to bite you when you resume your normal habits. Instead of following fad diets, try making permanent, sustainable lifestyle changes for forever weight loss and fitness.

Count Your Liquid Calories

What you drink is a part of what you eat. Many people, unaware of this, sip in all their excess calories through sodas, iced teas and cocktails. Alcohol and sugar-rich drinks are full of empty calories; they don't satisfy your hunger, and contribute to a range of health problems. For some, cutting back on these can easily save the 200–300 calories a day you need to start losing weight.

If you're thirsty, stick to water. If you really need something with flavor, try adding a splash of unsweetened fruit juice, or try flavored sparkling water or skim milk. Limit your alcohol consumption to one or two drinks on the weekend, and if you're eating out, order a small or kids' size soda, if you simply must indulge.

Eat Fresh

Health experts agree that snacking between meals is one of the biggest diet downfalls. That's when most people hit the vending machine, where there's not much fresh fruit to be had; instead, it's cookies, chips, or cakes, undoing all the good work of your healthy breakfast and lunch. Unhealthy snacks can be responsible for another 300–400 calories in the average person's diet, stalling weight loss progress and even adding weight despite healthy meals and exercise.

If you want to lose weight without dieting, though, you can turn your snack cravings from enemy to ally. Just stock up on fruit! A bowl of chopped, seasonal fruit has fewer calories than a candy bar, is more filling, and contains more nutrients. A glass of unsweetened, fresh juice can also be a tasty snack.

Additionally, be liberal with your vegetable portions at mealtime. Vegetables have the same healthy properties as fruit, and they go well with every main course you can think of. There are endless ways to prepare and eat vegetables, both fresh and cooked, so you can have a different side dish at every meal and never get bored.

Lean Proteins Are Key

Fad diets focus on gimmicks and extreme changes; they don't tell you about simple, sustainable lifestyle changes, like adding protein to your diet. Nuts, beans and lentils, lean meats, dairy, even peanut butter are all great protein sources. A small protein portion with every meal will keep you full and help prevent overeating.

If you apply these practical steps to lose weight without dieting, you'll find you have less space—and even desire—for junk food and processed sweets. Your waistline and overall health will benefit.

23

Lose Weight Fast with Muscle Building

While looking for the right method to lose weight fast, you've probably already been bombarded with information. There's plenty of conflicting and confusing theories out there, most from parties trying to tempt you into a product or service. There's no need to buy into a weight loss scheme or a $200 fitness DVD set. All you really need to do is lift weights.

More Muscle Means Faster Metabolism

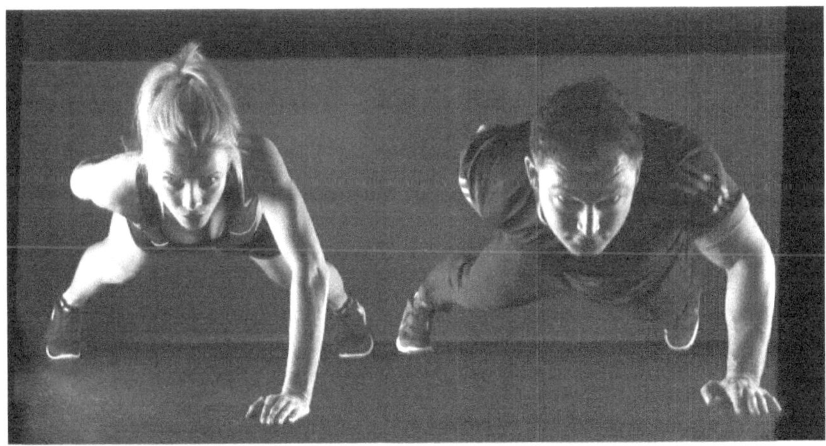

Your body has both fat and muscle, no matter how fit you are, and they have opposite effects on your metabolism, or the rate at which you burn calories. Fat slows the metabolic rate; muscle speeds it up. So the more muscle you have, the more calories you'll burn in a day, even while at rest. In combination with a healthy diet, you're well on your way to a lean, fit body. Here's where to start:

Your body consists of both fat and muscle, and they have opposite effects on your metabolism, which is the rate at which your body burns calories. While fat slows down your metabolic rate, muscle speeds it up. So, the more lean muscle you have, the more calories your body will burn in a day, even while at rest! Combine an enhanced metabolic rate with a controlled diet, and you have cracked the weight loss problem. However, once you have decided to embark on a muscle building program, you have to know the right way to do it.

Warm Up

A good warm-up session of fifteen to twenty minutes is important, to make sure your muscles have optimal range of motion and minimize the risk of injury. It should consist of five to ten minutes of light cardio, such as a brisk walk or slow jog, and a stretching circuit.

Posture

Posture is important in weight lifting. If your posture isn't correct, you'll be wasting your effort at best, and risking serious injury at worst. Consider hiring a trainer, at least for a few weeks, while you learn the basics.

Allow the Body to Adapt

Those massive weights in the corner look exciting, but they're not for you; at least, not yet. For the first few weeks, you need to give your muscles time to adapt to the additional work you're giving them. You shouldn't be lifting anything so heavy you're struggling to do a repetition. Limit each exercise to a single set of eight to ten reps each. Once your body gets used to this, you can add an extra set of each exercise.

The Necessity of Rest

Time spent outside of the gym is not necessarily wasted. Muscles adapt and grow in the period of rest following a workout, not during the workout itself. Make sure you give yourself a few days' rest each week, to give your body time to rebuild.

No 'Best Formula'

Rather, there is a best formula for success, but it's unique to you. Different techniques may all be equally effective; however, whatever method you choose, make sure to challenge your body with something new every two or three weeks. Add weight, vary your routine, or add a new exercise, but know that doing the same routine over and over will cause a plateau in your weight loss, once your body adjusts.

Finally, remember you'll only lose weight quickly and consistently if you follow a balanced diet plan. Don't starve yourself, though—you need to feed the machine.

24

Mental Training for Weight Loss: The Role Your Mind Plays in Helping You Lose Weight

For as long as humans have been self-aware, we've believed in the indomitable spirit of the mind. Few, however, have ever come close to measuring it in empirical terms. Despite a lack of unimpeachable evidence, we all have our own personal mind-over-matter stories. So, when we embark on a weight loss program, we plan for physical exercise and diet—should we include mental training as well? How would we even go about it? And would it be worth the effort? A study conducted by Harvard University may have some answers.

Hotel cleaning attendants lead a very active lifestyle. The nature of their work keeps them moving for several hours a day, and includes labor such as vacuuming, lifting, scrubbing, bending and stretching. Researchers wondered if the attendants knew the positive benefits of their job on their health. And, if they *were* made aware, would it enact any changes in their body, such as weight loss and lower blood pressure?

More than 80 cleaning attendants from seven different hotels were divided into two groups. The first group was educated on how many calories they burned as they went about their daily job responsibilities, and given handouts illustrating each activity and the amount of calories it burned.

On the other hand, the second group wasn't given this information, though they were informed of the benefits of exercising, the fact that their work was a great form of exercise and burned a lot of calories was kept from them.

Afterward, the groups were monitored regularly, and care was taken that none of the participants changed any of their lifestyle habits outside of work, such as diet, smoking or exercising, to make sure external factors didn't affect the results of the study. Even the workload of the participants was kept strictly constant.

The results were eye-opening, to say the least. People in the first group showed *significant* weight loss, decreased blood pressure, lower BMI (body mass index) and a more favorable waist-to-hip ratio. The second group, however, showed no improvement whatsoever.

Researchers believe the difference in results between the two groups is owed to what we can only describe as mental training for weight-loss—mind over matter. Since all other factors were kept constant, the only variable was awareness of their job's calorie-burning potential. As a result, the first group kept in mind the benefits of the activities they were performing throughout the day. Clearly, the brain is a powerful motivator.

The lesson is that it's not enough to simply go through the motions; you have to "believe it to achieve it," to quote a motivational poster. So, as you digest your healthy meal, try to envision it feeding your growing muscles. While working out, imagine what your body will feel like when it's slender. Picture the muscles working under your skin, and the fat oozing out of your pores and evaporating like sweat. Be mindful and aware of all you do, and it could very well speed you down the path to success.

25

Natural Foods That Help Burn Belly Fat

While some articles and experts preach that nature (or science) have produced miracle fat-burning foods, others are quick to point out that what really counts is your overall calories in/calories out ratio. In fact, most dieticians dismiss the supposed fat-burning properties of natural foods and herbal concoctions as irresponsible myths. Who do we believe? Are there any natural foods that burn belly fat, or not?

The truth is that there are no foods that *directly* burn belly fat. When physical trainers and dieticians say what counts is calories, they're right. But there are many factors which affect your actual metabolic rate, or how many calories you burn in a resting state. One of these is diet. There are foods which promote the production of the right hormones and chemicals to speed your metabolism and accelerate fat-burning. In other words, these foods won't burn fat, but they'll help *you* burn fat.

Cinnamon

Cinnamon is one of nature's most powerful spices when it comes to fat loss, and that's because it helps control your blood sugar level. A study published in Diabetes Care, a medical journal, shows that consuming 3–6 grams of cinnamon per day can reduce fasting blood glucose levels by up to 29%. Cinnamon also helps maintain high insulin sensitivity, and together, these factors directly boost your body's ability to fight fat. This extremely versatile spice can be added to cereal, dessert, fruit, main courses, and even your coffee.

Broccoli and Cauliflower

In modern urban life, you're constantly exposed to harmful chemicals known as xenoestrogens, due to environmental pollution and chemical compounds used in food. Studies have shown that these chemicals promote the storage of excess fat in your body. It's impossible to escape xenoestrogens—they're everywhere—but by consuming cruciferous vegetables such as broccoli, cabbage and cauliflower, you can fight off the harmful fat-storing effects of this chemical. These greens are some of nature's most effective fat-burning foods.

Nuts

With their high calorie and fat content, you may be surprised to see nuts on a list of foods which burn belly fat. All fat is not created equal, though, and nuts contain plenty of the healthy kind, as well as protein, antioxidants, vitamins and minerals. Protein-rich foods fight hunger and help maintain your body's muscle mass, both essential for weight loss and maintenance. Their micronutrients also help your body's production of fat-burning hormones. Whatever kind of nuts you prefer, a handful a day won't do you any harm. You can also try peanut or other nut butters, for a sweet, creamy treat.

Keep in mind that the fat-burning effect of these foods is *indirect;* they're not magic potions. You still need to make good choices in terms of diet and exercise, but if you complement your efforts with these foods, you'll see better, faster results.

26

6 Essential Muscle Training Tips to Lose Weight Fast

In order to lose weight fast, exercise should be an essential part of your routine. If you have time, weight and resistance training will speed up your metabolism and keep excess weight at bay. You'll also feel more energetic, and better about your sleeker, more powerful body. Before you begin to incorporate weight training into your weight loss routine, though, there are a few things you should know:

1. Muscle Building vs Muscle Toning

When most people think of muscle building, they picture professional bodybuilders with unnaturally bulging muscles. Don't worry; that won't happen to you, not unless you want it to. There's a big difference between *toning* muscles and building *bulky* muscles. If you want to be strong and have a lean, athletic look at the same time, then muscle toning belongs in your routine. Muscle toning involves resistance exercises which use body weight, like squats and pushups, or doing more repetitions with lighter weights. If you'd prefer to bulk up, go with heavier weights and lower reps.

2. The Right Weight Loss Strategy

While you're losing weight, the emphasis should be on toning rather than bulking up, because losing weight fast requires consuming less calories than you burn in a day. Provided you eat healthy, you can tone your muscles simultaneously. Building muscles, however, requires you to consume more calories than you burn, to "feed" them. That's not compatible with fat loss, so focusing on toning will both build the lean muscle base you need to raise your metabolic rate, and sculpt that lean, firm body you're working toward.

3. Warm Up and Cool Down

It's very important to warm up all the muscles you'll be exercising in any given session with light cardio and stretching, to help prevent injury. Light stretching is also necessary after exercise as well. This is known as a cool down, and helps your muscles recover faster by flushing lactic acid, a byproduct of muscle activity and the culprit of your morning-after soreness, from your body.

4. Flexibility

Some exercise systems, like yoga, emphasize flexibility and posture, and make an excellent addition to a weight training routine. The more you improve your flexibility, the better your muscles' range of motion, and the less likely you are to injure yourself.

5. Maintaining Good Form

While you're doing any exercise, it's important to maintain good form and posture, but it's especially important during weight training. Many people focus on hitting a certain weight or repetition goal. But you'll get more value from doing a single repetition with a lower weight correctly than you will doing it incorrectly ten times with heavier weights. You also increase your risk of injury when doing exercises improperly. There's a right way for a good reason, so seek the advice of a trainer or gym staff, especially if you're just starting out.

6. Training the Entire Body

If you want to get lean and fit, you need to train your entire body. Not all at once, though. If you focus on your arms and shoulders one day, work your legs the next, and your abs the day after that. And don't forget to give yourself rest days—muscles are built in the time after, not during, your weight-lifting sessions.

Why Racquetball is a Great Way to Lose Weight

When people think of a weight loss plan, the first thing that comes to mind is going to a gym or adopting a rigorous diet. Since both of these are intense commitments, most people never quite get around to taking the initiative, so, of course, they never lose weight. If you've felt the same way, and are ready for a change, perhaps it's time to consider some interesting and fun ways to lose weight, such as racquetball.

Why Racquetball?

Racquetball is very similar to squash, requiring quick turns, speed, and agility. As soon as you've hit the ball, you have to immediately get back to your position to prepare for its return. As you can imagine, this really gets your heart racing! Racquetball is an excellent cardiovascular exercise, and also helps improve your flexibility, muscular strength, and endurance.

You might be thinking racquetball is only for people who are already in good shape, but that's not true at all. Even if you only play within your fitness and skill level, you'll still reap all the cardiovascular and muscular benefits. Remember, *every* exercise or sport is meant to be performed only within your physical capabilities. Try to find a partner who's roughly at your level, or, if competition isn't your cup of tea, you can even play alone.

How Many Calories Does It Burn?

If you want to get straight to the hard figures and find out exactly how effective racquetball is for weight loss, we've got some good news for you. According to the Mayo Clinic, a 160-pound person can burn approximately 511 calories playing an hour of moderate-intensity racquetball. The number goes up to 637 calories for a 200-pound person, and 763 calories for a 240-pound individual. Considering it's just a 'moderate' intensity exercise, those numbers stack up pretty well! And when you play regularly, your muscles will become stronger, boosting your resting metabolic rate.

Racquetball and Weight Loss – What the Numbers Say

Taking the numbers further, if you play racquetball for an hour three to four times a week, you could lose 12–13 pounds in three months! Other people go through a lot of suffering to lose that much weight. Of course, you'll only successfully lose weight if you control your diet, too. That doesn't mean you have to rigorously count calories; just eat healthy, avoid processed foods, and you'll be on the right track.

Lots of Fun!

One major advantage of racquetball is that, since it's a sport rather than an exercise, it won't get monotonous. Going to the gym means suffering through an hour of exercise, watching the clock, just waiting for it to be over. A sport, on the other hand, is *fun,* and you'll find yourself motivated to maintain a regular routine in the long run. If you plan to embark on a weight loss journey through racquetball, just be sure to stretch for ten minutes before and after your game, to avoid injuries.

27

Can a Massage Help You Lose Weight?

According to qualified medical experts, massage doesn't play a direct role in weight loss. However, it has quite a few *indirect* weight loss benefits, and makes a great addition to any weight loss plan.

First, it's important to understand that weight loss only happens when you burn more calories than you consume. A calorie deficit forces your body to break down fat reserves for energy. To achieve a calorie deficit, you need to follow an exercise regime and control your diet. Surprisingly, massage can help you achieve both.

Massage and Stress Reduction

One of the major causes of overeating and bingeing on high-calorie, high-sugar foods is stress. When people are overworked, or under emotional or mental pressure, they seek relief in food, which invariably leads to a calorie surplus and weight gain. Massage is known to help relax the body and bring down stress levels, by stimulating the parasympathetic nervous system. The resulting state of overall relaxation may help you cope with pressures, and you might not need to resort to food for comfort.

Massage and Exercise

When you begin an exercise regime, or intensify an existing one, you'll most likely find yourself dealing with muscle pain, soreness, or injuries. Massage has been proven to stretch and relax muscles, reduce soreness, and improve circulation. This improves your flexibility, endurance, and recovery, reducing the chances of injury and helping you work out harder for longer.

Improved Blood Circulation

Another crucial connection between massage and weight loss is improved circulation, as we already mentioned. Improved circulation means your body's mechanism for feeding oxygen and nutrients to your muscles and removing waste products is improved. Your body will perform more efficiently during exercise, and you'll be able to exercise longer, burning more calories.

Improved Skin Elasticity

When people lose a lot of weight rapidly, especially if they're older or have been overweight for a long time, they often experience loose, saggy skin. Massage helps the skin remain supple and encourages it to tighten as you lose weight, helping you achieve the toned, taut look you desire.

More Efficient Digestive System

Massage has also been known to improve the function and efficiency of the digestive system, by facilitating the breakdown of food and waste, which could prevent the body from accumulating excess fat. Though many people have experienced this personally, it's important to note there's a lack of conclusive evidence to back this assertion.

Again, massage makes an excellent complement to a weight loss plan; it shouldn't be your only strategy. But as a part of a responsible diet and exercise regime, it can help you reach your goals—and, if nothing else, it's a great, calorie-free way to treat yourself for all your hard work!

28

Losing Weight with Zumba – It's Fun!

People dance, or people exercise. The first is done for fun and creative satisfaction; the second, for weight loss and fitness. What if you could combine the two, and reap the benefits of both? It might not be the most revolutionary idea, but with Zumba, the latest dance-exercise craze catching on all over the world, the combination becomes more fun and effective than ever before.

What Is It?

Zumba is the brainchild of aerobics instructor Alberto Perez. It involves a combination of dance rhythms of varying intensities, borrowed from Latin dances and set to Latin music. The classes alternate between intervals of fast-paced, vigorous dancing and slower, more relaxed movements. Typically, classes are an hour long, and the music plays non-stop, meaning there's no period of complete rest. In other words, your body is burning calories for the entire hour!

How Many Calories Does Zumba Burn?

For those looking to lose weight, the number of calories expended by Zumba is one of the most attractive features. An hour of Zumba can burn between 500–800 calories, depending on your body weight and fitness levels; for example, a 150-pound person can expect to burn about 535 calories during an hour of Zumba, compared to 420 calories for the same period of moderate swimming, less than 500 for racquetball, and 680 calories for jogging.

How Popular and Genuine is Zumba for Weight Loss?

Zumba might seem to have popped up spontaneously, but its success isn't random. Since its creation in 2001, this dance-exercise combination has spread to over 110 countries and captivated ten million people. All instructors are fully-trained, and must be licensed by the Zumba academy in the US. There are several types of Zumba classes, customized for those of different fitness levels and dance abilities. So, whether you're a beginner, or someone who's already a fit, competent dancer, you have something to gain—or lose—from Zumba.

By alternating intense spells of aerobic dance and periods of light movement, Zumba incorporates the principles of interval training. Interval training is known to burn more calories than steady-paced exercises, dancing, or aerobic, and accelerates fitness and weight loss. Not only does Zumba burn calories, it also tones muscles, boosts metabolic rate, and improves flexibility.

Zumba is great for weight loss, but, perhaps just as importantly, it's a lot of fun, which helps you stay motivated and interested, and keeps you from watching the clock during your hour of exercise.

Due to its unique combination of effective fitness and fun, the Zumba Academy advertises cases of people who've lost up to one hundred pounds, with Zumba as their only cardiovascular exercise. So if you're looking for a fun, interesting way to lose weight, check out your neighborhood class.

29

Weight Loss with Raw Food Diet – Is It Sustainable and Beneficial?

Far too many diets market themselves as a sure-shot way to lose a ton of weight fast. But the question you should always ask is whether a diet is sustainable and beneficial, as well. Of course, you can lose weight by abusing your body with an incomplete diet, and risk serious malnutrition. But this strategy isn't sustainable. It ruins your health, and the results are fleeting—the weight always comes back. Which category does the raw food diet fall into?

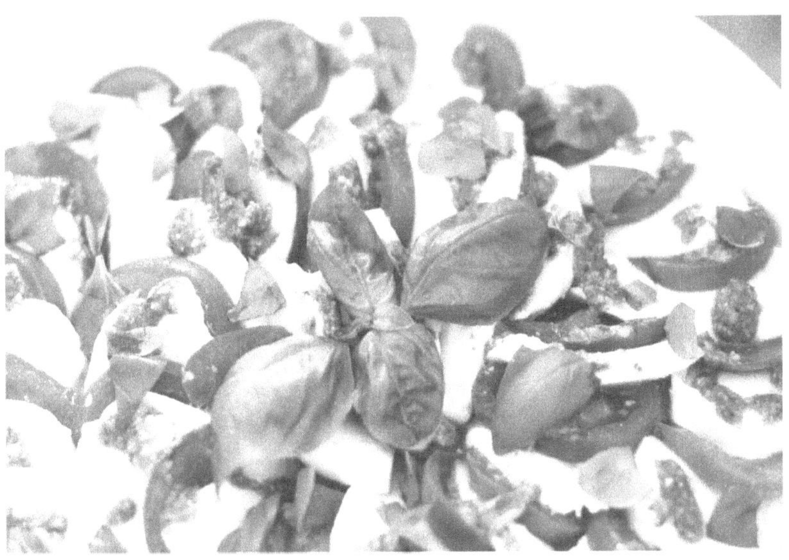

Not a Restrictive Diet

One of the best things about the raw food diet is that it's not severely restrictive. Yes, you're limited to raw food, but 'raw food' covers an immense amount of variety, and all you have to do is eat balanced portions. As far as quantity goes, there's no restriction—since fruits and vegetables have an extremely low calorie-to-mass ratio, you can eat as much as you need to feel full, without worrying about excess calories.

One of the Best Weight Loss Diets

The raw-food diet is as near to a fail-proof method as you'll ever find for weight loss. You phase out all high-calorie rich meals and processed sugars, substituting them with fiber and nutrient-rich raw foods, which are much lower in calories. With the exception of nuts, some seeds, and bananas, it's difficult to find a natural, raw food that's rich in calories. If you're overweight, you could lose 6–9 pounds a month on the raw food diet, without putting yourself through torturous weight loss methods.

Is Weight Loss the Only Benefit of the Raw Food Diet?

Not at all. Uncooked foods are richer in vitamins and minerals than their cooked counterparts, offering numerous benefits, like peak organ performance, hormonal balance, radiant skin and strong bones. A raw food diet also detoxifies the body, and keeps the digestive system in great shape.

If you're following an exercise regime as well, it's important not to ignore your protein needs. Sprouted grains and lentils, as well as nuts, are great raw sources of protein.

100% Raw?

If you went 100% raw, there'd be no harm done—it's how nature intended. However, it's just not practical in modern society. If you can maintain a 50%–75% raw food diet, that's more than sufficient. Many people maintain this for a short period of time to lose weight and detoxify the body, so a 4–12 week period may be enough.

30

How to Lose 10 Pounds Fast and Easy – So How About a Quick Fix Diet?

No one is happy being overweight or obese; it's neither desirable nor healthy. So most people, if they want to lose ten pounds, think the faster they lose that weight, the better. This is the sort of attitude that drives people to drastic 'crash' diets. There are other motivators too, such as getting in shape for an upcoming beach holiday or wedding. But drastic weight reduction isn't healthy, and crash diets are never effective in the long run.

What is a Crash Diet?

Essentially, a 'crash' or quick-fix diet is any severely restrictive diet, and often involves fasting. It's a fast path to a short-term weight loss goal, and many people even go on crash diets knowing they're risking their health. Even the diet program curators add health disclaimers, warning people against practicing them for longer than a week or ten days. But an unhealthy diet is still unhealthy even in the short-term.

Slow Metabolism

If you want to lose those ten pounds and keep them off, you have to understand the relationship of your metabolism to your body. When your body sees a drastic reduction of fuel, it goes into starvation mode, preparing itself to survive a famine. Rather than burning calories, it stores them as fat, the equivalent of a savings account for a rainy day. This metabolic slowdown can spell disaster for your health; when you return to a normal diet, your body is no longer capable of burning even a maintenance level of calories. That excess weight will come right back, and you might even end up heavier than you were when you started.

Loss of Fluids, Not Fat

This might surprise you, but a lot of the weight you lose through a crash diet is fluids rather than fat. The numbers on the scale might be different, and you might even see a difference in your waistline, but at the end of the day, you've wasted effort you might have spent on a legitimate weight loss plan.

Cravings and Depression

People on crash diets often experience intense food cravings, loss of concentration, and even serious depression, so much so that it's almost considered a part of the diet experience. It's not easy for your body and mind to handle such a drastic shock, and your body tries to warn you of the danger by using these symptoms as alarm bells. Your body views a rapid loss of ten pounds cause for serious concern; you should, too.

Losing Out on Vital Nutrients

When you go on a severely restrictive diet, such as a liquid-only or extreme low-carb diet, the body loses out on vital nutrients, which can cause damage to the liver, kidney, or heart. It's more than just your metabolism at stake—it's your lifelong health.

A Strong Temptation

Those who promote crash diets are familiar with these risks, and this is why they only recommend their diets for a short period. That doesn't change the fact that they're not healthy, period. The only reason crash diets still exist is thanks to those who simply can't resist the temptation of losing ten pounds virtually overnight.

Your best chance is to make sustainable, healthy lifestyle changes. Adopt a well-rounded, nutritious, and wholesome diet, and incorporate exercise into your routine. Your metabolism gets a boost, your overall health improves, and your weight loss will be steady, consistent, and lasting. Six months down the road, when your friend has already gained back all the weight she lost on that trendy crash diet, you'll have a reason to be proud of yourself.

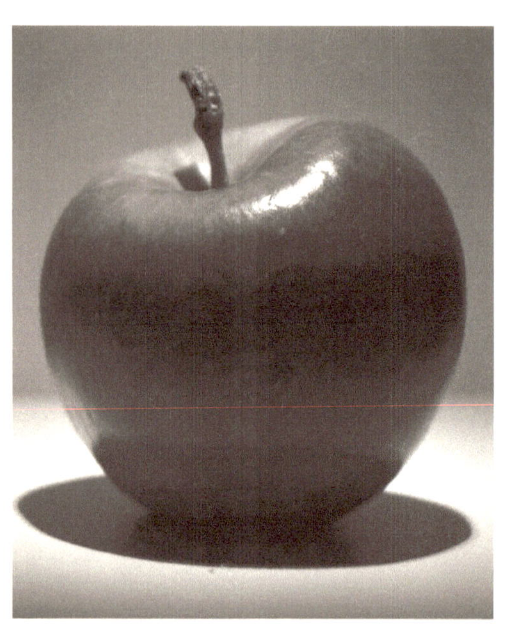

31

Portion Control for Weight Loss: Have Your Favorite Snacks and Still Lose Weight

Consistent weight loss is virtually impossible without some form of diet control. Unfortunately, people get carried away by the temptation of short-term results and fall for drastic diet measures, which are unsustainable and counterproductive in the long run. It doesn't have to be that difficult; one of the most practical and effective diet strategies is portion control, especially regarding snacks.

Be Practical

It's simple—in order to lose weight, you need to consume fewer calories than you burn. Well, the concept is simple; unfortunately, growing portion sizes and calorie-rich food temptations make it harder than it sounds.

Some people try to go cold-turkey, replacing all their favorite snacks with fruits and vegetables, but this strategy generally only leads to frustration and failure. You'll be much more successful by enjoying your favorite snacks in moderation—in other words, exercising portion control.

Buy Small Packs

Your home is where you have most control over what you eat, so be responsible. Stop buying big bags of chips, cookies, wafers, and other calorie-rich processed goodies.

If these temptations are available within reach, you're going to end up reaching for them, so don't set yourself up for failure.

Buy small packages, or immediately split the big package into individual portions and seal them up in a sandwich baggie. This is a great way to beat the psychological aspects of weight loss—you'll stop eating when the portion is gone, not when your brain gets the delayed signal of fullness from your stomach, and you'll be less likely to reach for two portions, when you know one is all you need.

Read Nutrition Labels

Before you divide your spoils, read the nutritional information, so you actually know how big a portion of your snack is. The nutritional label will tell you what constitutes a portion size, and also gives you a breakdown of vitamins, minerals, sodium, and sugar percentages, based on a 2,000 calorie diet. It might become tedious to count 27 crackers out into each of ten different bags, though, so consider investing in a kitchen scale—it'll help you manage your portions for all your food, not just your snacks.

Stock Healthy Snacks

You don't have to replace all your snacks with healthier fare, but you should replace some. Make sure they're properly placed, too—a jar of nuts should be in easier reach than the cookies, and the fruit should hold pride of place in the front of the refrigerator.

Exercise Control During TV Hours

Here's another reason to measure out your portions beforehand: some of the worst diet disasters happen in front of the TV, where there's a tendency to mindlessly shovel down chips or cookies while relaxed and distracted by their favorite show. You can undo a week's hard work in a single hour of mindless TV munching, so be sure to watch those portions!

Eat Slowly

As we mentioned, it takes your brain a while to realize your stomach is full, so make sure you don't wolf down your snack—you can overfill your stomach before you even realize it. Your snack should be a treat, not a staple, so slow down and make it last! When you eat slowly, you'll be satisfied with less. And if you find yourself still hungry after the last bite, grab some fruit or nuts to top off the tank, instead of another cookie.

32

Why Beginners Lose Their Motivation
Instead of Their Weight

Right after New Year's, interest in fitness swells to its highest annual peak. Suddenly, everyone wants to lose weight and get fit. Gyms find themselves bursting at the seams. Unfortunately, though, this storm fades as rapidly as it sweeps in, and by the time February rolls around, all that enthusiasm is virtually gone. It's a trend experts are well aware of, and they have some advice for beginners. By being aware of the reasons why people jump the fitness ship, you might be able to protect yourself from a similar fate.

Planning

If your resolution is to lose weight and look fitter, but all you do is head to the gym with no goal more concrete than this broad abstraction, you're not going to last long. Having specific plans and goals, and working out a clear schedule to achieve them, is extremely important, if you want to maintain your motivation and enthusiasm.

To begin with, find your path. Are you going to invest in workout equipment? Take up running? Join the neighborhood martial arts dojo? Once you've decided, you need to map out specific and achievable short-term goals, and a plan to achieve them. You'll find a wealth of resources out there to help you, like fitness trainers, running clubs, books, and DVDs.

Too Enthusiastic, Too Intense, Too Fatigued

Inspired by your goals, you may be tempted to be too ambitious, too soon. You might squeeze in too many sessions, or work at an intensity beyond your capabilities, or both. But when beginners get in over their heads, they end up with aches, pains, and fatigue. Delayed Onset of Muscular Soreness (DOMS) is a common phenomenon among beginners. And the minute you start dreading your workouts, or skipping them because you're too sore, the end of your New Year's resolution is near. Stick with a steady pace, and don't push yourself too hard, at least for the first few weeks.

20-Minute Sessions

A contributor to DOMS, and fitness failure in general, may be the mindset that if you don't get in at least an hour of exercise during a session, you might as well not work out at all. In fact, the opposite is true; most experts now believe a relatively intense 20 minute session is more productive than a moderate hour-long session.

Overeating

No weight loss article is complete without a mention of food and diet. As it relates to exercise, you need to be careful that you don't overeat after working out. Naturally, your body will demand food after exercise, but be careful not to counteract potential weight loss by putting all the calories you just burned right back in. Stay away from calorie-rich food, and try some fresh fruit or a handful of nuts to quell your hunger pangs.

33

5 Most Effective Tips for Your Weight Loss Workout

If you've decided on consistent exercise as your path to achieving your weight loss goals, you're on the right track. Now, all you need to do is find out how to get the maximum benefit out of your workouts.

1. Choose an Exercise you Enjoy

If you want to stick to your plan beyond the first few months, this is crucial. When you come across a miraculous weight loss story, you'll invariably find that the person in question fell in love with their exercise of choice. Your weight loss workout needs to be interesting enough that you'd want to do it even if you *weren't* trying to lose weight. Try bicycling, martial arts, yoga, dance, or any of the numerous activities that combine fitness with fun. Don't feel like a failure if one doesn't work out for you—just try another. And remember, you don't have to commit to just one!

2. High Intensity, Short Duration

Exercise doesn't have to be a long, drawn-out effort in order to work for weight loss. In fact, if you continue exercising when you're fatigued, you're not really going to get much out of it (except maybe an injury). High intensity/short duration weight loss workouts are much more effective, efficient and practical. You burn more calories per minute, and build muscles more quickly, which will boost your metabolism. This approach works with both cardiovascular and weight training workouts.

3. Build a Base First

Without a foundation, a structure will collapse; this applies to your body, too. So before you turn up the heat on your workouts, be sure to give your body at least a month to adapt to its new challenges. If you're starting off with jogging or cycling, the first month should involve moderate-to-low intensity efforts. If you're getting breathless, you're working too hard. For jogging, a great beginner's plan is the Mayo Clinic's couch-to-5k program. Similarly, if you're doing any kind of weight training, you should be concentrating on form, rather than how much weight is on your bar. Gradually build up to a level where your body can handle higher intensities. After that, the sky's the limit!

4. Don't Do the Same Thing Every Day

Once your body adapts to a certain workout, it becomes more efficient at completing it, requiring less calories during the effort and stagnating your weight loss goals. Keep your body guessing by giving it new challenges; that's the only way to keep climbing the ladder to fitness and weight loss success. Rather than running the same route every day, incorporate some higher-speed intervals one day, some uphill running on another, and strengthening exercises on the weekend.

5. Don't Do It Every Day

Rest is crucial for your body; it's when muscles repair, adapt, and grow. Without enough rest, you also expose yourself to injury and physical and mental fatigue, making your weight loss workout unsustainable. Ideally, your body should have 1–3 days of complete rest per week, depending on how hard you're working.

34

3 Effective Facial Exercises to Lose Face Fat Fast and Get a Lean, Firm and Young Face

Your face is the only part of your body that's always visible, and always reveals the state of your health, for better or for worse. You can't disguise facial fat with makeup, either—but you can get rid of it fast, with discipline and exercise. You should begin to see a marked difference within weeks.

How Facial Exercises Help

Weight loss isn't a process you can restrict to just one area of the body. In order to lose weight, you have to burn more calories than you consume; then your body will burn its fat reserves for energy.

However, with specific facial exercises, you can tone the muscles of your face, giving it a firmer, leaner look, and a more defined structure. In combination with a weight loss regime, your face will be looking slimmer in no time.

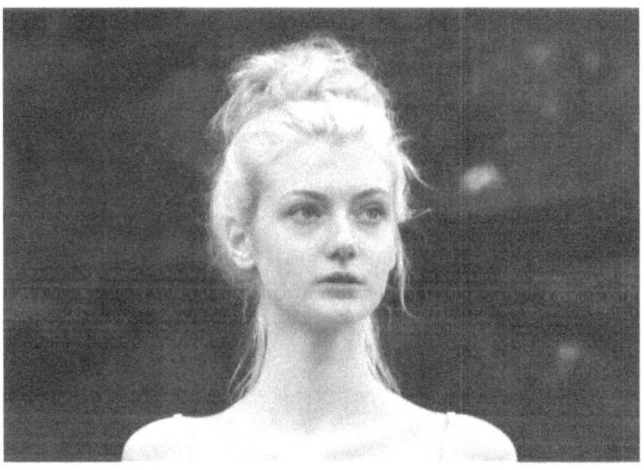

1. The Smiling Exercise

Smiling is one of the most natural facial expressions, and a great facial exercise, too! First, smile as widely as you possibly can. Holding your smile, turn your head slowly, from left to center, then right to center, then release the smile gently, keeping your movements smooth. Repeat these ten times, twice a day, to tone your cheek muscles.

2. Open Your Mouth Wide

This exercise targets that hateful double chin. Start off by opening your mouth as wide as it will go, stretching your jaw as much as possible. Hold for a few seconds, and then slowly release the strain. Repeat ten times, three times a day.

3. Blow Air

This is an excellent exercise to correct frown lines and tone your chin and cheeks. Curl your lips inward over your teeth, open your mouth very slightly, and blow air from your lungs into your mouth, just enough so the areas around your mouth, but not your cheeks, puff out. Hold for six to eight seconds, and then release the air. Repeat this twice a day, ten times each.

Remember, your facial muscles are like any other muscles in the body. With exercise and toning, they'll get stronger and have a leaner, firmer appearance. Just don't do these exercises in public—you might get some funny looks!

You Need a General Exercise Regime

As we mentioned, these exercises will help tone your facial muscles, but you won't actually lose face fat. For that, you need a comprehensive exercise plan, with calorie-burning cardiovascular and muscle-toning exercises for the major muscle groups of the body.

For cardio, if you're pressed for time, brisk walking or jogging for 20–30 minutes will fit the bill; you can even incorporate walking into your daily routine.

Muscle toning improves your metabolism, so you'll be able to burn more calories at rest, helping you lose both face and body fat quickly. There are several excellent muscle-toning exercises that can be done in your living room, with no equipment needed.

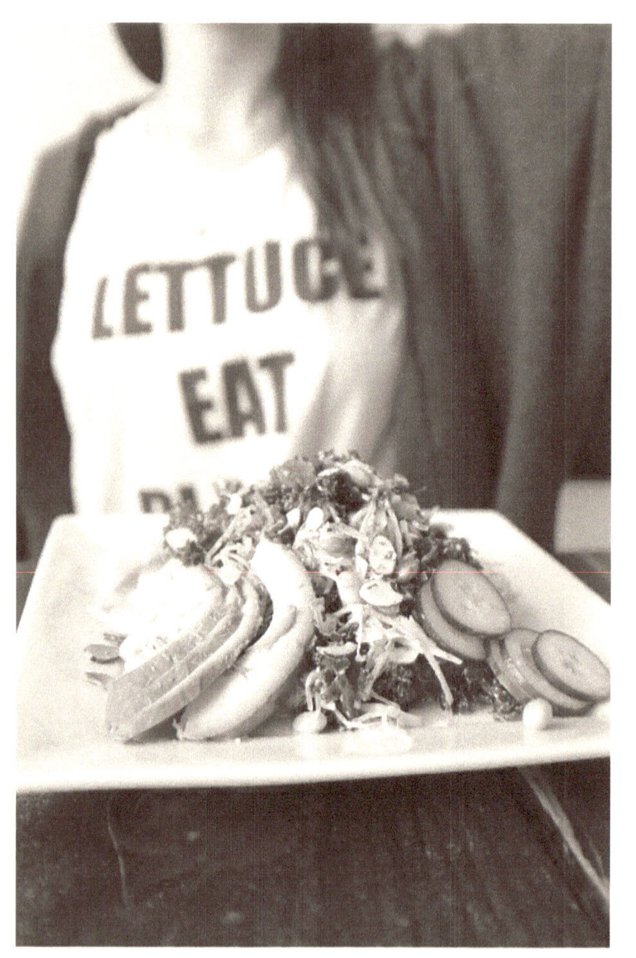
LETTUCE
EAT

35

5 Essential Tips to Follow the Raw Food Diet for Weight Loss

The raw food diet has become very popular as a weight loss strategy. Many people, however, are frightened away just by the name. 'Raw food diet' calls to mind a person munching on carrot sticks and sprouts all day long. It feels primitive, restrictive, and radical, and almost impossible to practice. Rest assured, though, that there's nothing primitive about the raw food diet.

Phase In the Diet

If you plan to just wake up one morning and begin your 100% raw food diet, you're setting yourself up for failure; you'll simply frustrate and intimidate yourself in a matter of days, if not hours. Not to mention your digestive system won't be equipped to handle this sudden dietary change, and you'll probably end up with stomach upset. It's a much better idea to phase the diet in gradually. Start by including raw food snacks (nuts and fruits), and substituting fruits for processed sweets when you have a sugar craving. Include raw foods into your meals, too, like a salad for dinner or a smoothie for breakfast. Next, replace one cooked meal with a completely raw one every day. Once your body is used to handling raw food on a regular basis, make the switch.

Not 100% Raw

But bear in mind that raw doesn't mean 100% raw. It's virtually impossible for anyone to practice a completely raw food diet for weight loss. Most people who successfully follow this diet plan stay at about 75% raw. The other 25% covers social occasions where cooked foods dominate, and the occasional treat, as well as certain regular exceptions.

These exceptions can include certain extras you may decide to include in your diet for health reasons, and there's nothing wrong with that. Many people, for instance, continue to use soy milk to meet their protein requirements.

A Lot More than Smoothies and Salads

If you thought a raw food diet consisted only of smoothies and salads, you'd be surprised to find the amount of variety available. Even with run-of-the-mill ingredients, people have come up with some remarkably creative recipes and alternatives for 'regular' food items. For example, you can make your own 'nut milk,' at home, or even raw cheese.

Go Organic

If you're going raw, this is a crucial tip. After all, you don't want to fill your body with deadly commercial pesticides. With vegan and raw food diets becoming more popular, however, organic fruits and vegetables aren't difficult to come by. The grocery store isn't your only option; you can find a farmer's market even in the middle of a big city, or join a co-op for a delivery of fresh vegetables every week.

Have a Plan

It's best to start with a four-week raw diet weight loss plan to begin. See how your body reacts, and how much progress you make. Then you can begin another four-week cycle, or extend it to a six- or twelve-week plan.

Bear in mind that the raw food diet is not the only healthy diet plan for weight loss. Many people find that it doesn't suit them or their lifestyle, or it doesn't make them happy. If you're one of them, don't worry—just try something else! The most important thing is not to give up.

36

The Lightest Indian Meals for Weight Watchers

Several weight watchers and weight loss aspirants choose to adopt an Indian vegetarian diet for weight loss. The advantages of the Indian diet are numerous – it is great in taste and rich in fiber; there is variety in cooking and preparation; the vegetables retain their nutritive value; and the cooking is light in calories. Here are some of the lightest Indian preparations that should be the staple for weight watchers.

Simple Meal: Dal, Vegetable Dish and Chapatti

One of the most distinct features of Indian cooking is its use of curried lentil and legume preparations known collectively as *dal*. Dal is rich in natural proteins, light in calories and filling. It is also a great source of some vital micronutrients. A simple traditional meal consists of two main dishes a dal and a vegetable recipe – served with a dry flat bread prepared from whole wheat flour, known as chapatti. This simple meal provides you with protein, fiber and healthy carbohydrates, and if you prepare it the right way, it is also light in calories. Avoid the use of butter and clarified butter (*ghee*), and try to use cooking techniques that involve minimal oil (covered in another article).

Raita as Accompaniment

Yoghurt is one of the major ingredients in Indian cooking and one of the country's most popular side dishes. Its cool flavor complements local spices and preparations styles really well. If it is prepared from reduced-fat milk, it is a great protein source, light in calories and very healthy. In other words, yoghurt is excellent for weight watchers. *Raita* is an Indian yoghurt preparation, consisting of several different vegetables and a range of mild local spices. Cucumber raita, onion and tomato raita, and potato raita are all popular in Indian households. Raita can be served as an accompaniment with any Indian meal, and it goes particularly well with the simple meal idea suggested above.

Khichdi

Khichdi is an Indian rice porridge that is common to several Indian cuisines. It is essentially a one dish meal, consisting of rice, dal and yoghurt blended together. It brings together all the benefits of these three food items, forming nothing less than a nutrition powerhouse (especially if you use unrefined rice). It is low in calories, rich in proteins, keeps you full and satisfied, and with its carbohydrate content, provides you with sustained energy release.

Indian Salads

Most people don't associate salads with Indian cooking, but that is a real mistake. Indians make a range of salads, and most of them are light and rich in fiber, proteins and complex carbohydrates. Sprouts salads are the best known of all Indian salads, and form a great breakfast item. Sprouted legumes form the main ingredient, and they are whipped together with chopped onions, tomatoes, cucumber, peanuts and potato. The special flavor comes from a combination of salt, lemon juice and local spices. This is a very versatile recipe, and you can vary the ingredients according to taste.

Bear in mind that these are only a few examples from several light Indian meals for weight watchers. There are a range of other dishes, especially from the Bengali and South Indian cuisines, that are perfectly suited for people who are out to lose weight. Do browse some of the other articles on the site for more information!

37

Boot Camps for Weight Loss – Fitness Phenomenon or Overrated Fad?

People are always on the lookout for new and exciting exercises to lose weight; for most, a morning jog or walk just doesn't cut it. And unless you're excited about your exercise routine, you won't be able to find the initiative to incorporate it into your lifestyle.

There are a lot of new weight loss workouts advertised on the market, targeted at this demographic. One of them is the idea of military-style "boot camps" for weight loss. This trend is gaining momentum in the UK and US, especially among people for whom exercise is a challenge.

A Fun Way to Lose Weight

Weight loss boot camps are adapted from military training regimes. Don't let that scare you away, though; boot camps are actually a lot of fun, since they bring people of diverse backgrounds and fitness levels together in an interactive and friendly team setup. Sure, there's the physical challenge, but there are also exciting games, good food, and the prospect of engaging social interaction. You'll make friends with like-minded people, and help each other push beyond your boundaries.

Flexible and Good for Everyone

The instructors are trained fitness experts, who adapt each person's workload according to their individual fitness levels, capacity, and objectives. With most boot camp companies, you can choose from a variety of packages, from an early-bird boot camp session, to weekend boot camp outings, and even boot camp vacations. There aren't many other exercise systems which offer such a unique combination of group atmosphere and flexibility.

The Benefits

The workouts involve a combination of cardiovascular and muscle-strengthening exercises, disguised as fun tasks with specific goals to achieve. During a boot camp session, you'll give your entire body a serious workout, burn a truckload of calories, and strengthen muscles you probably haven't used in a long time. Many people have reportedly lost 5–9 pounds during a seven-day boot camp session, and considering the comprehensive emphasis on healthy eating and exercise, these claims don't seem exaggerated. The best part is that boot camps can be adapted to every fitness level and age group, so no one gets left out.

Possible Drawbacks

The fact is that boot camp is very intensive. It might not suit people who've been sedentary for a long time and want to ease into a fitness routine; it can even be intimidating for people not used to exercise.

Additionally, boot camps are short-term programs. Even if you lose a lot of weight, you'll gain it right back if you slip into old habits after the session. Make sure you heed the diet and exercise tips your boot camp instructor gives you, and make sustainable lifestyle changes after the camp is over.

The final verdict? Boot camps are extremely effective for weight loss, but you'll only reap the benefits long-term if you implement good habits after the session is complete.

38

6 Celebrity Weight Loss Diet Secrets Revealed

Most female celebrities are popular for two reasons—their beauty, and their figure. A lot of women use celebrities as role models, and hope to achieve a similarly slim and sexy body. But have you ever stopped to wonder how they actually do it? Not all celebrities follow a sustainable diet; in fact, most are notorious for their bizarre and downright silly fad diets that help them drop pounds within days. Don't believe me? Take a look at some of the more popular celebrity weight loss diets.

1. Master Cleanse Diet

This is one of the more popular fad diets claiming to help you lose weight fast. Sure, an American artist, actress and fashion designer dropped about twenty pounds on this diet, but who wouldn't, if they were consuming nothing more than a concoction of lemon juice, maple syrup, and cayenne pepper?

2. Baby Food Diet

Come on, now! You're going to dip into your baby's food? This is one of those celebrity weight loss diets which sounds silly from the word *go*. So, put down your baby's bowl and look for a more grown-up solution for weight loss!

3. Eat Like a Bird Fad

Taking inspiration from birds? Why not, considering that very few birds lose sleep over weight loss issues, and they're always in form. Plus, they can fly! That seems to be an English singer/songwriter's reasoning, as she sincerely champions the virtues of eating like a bird. The secret behind her svelte body is a diet of soya beans, strawberries, lettuce, and a gross shake of algae and seaweed. What bird is she using for inspiration, I wonder?

4. Grapefruit Oil Diet

One Hollywood actress believes in sniffing grapefruit oil to keep her figure. Why, exactly? Well, "experts" in "liver psychology" argue that the scent of grapefruit releases a secret message, propelling the liver into action attacking fat deposits in your body with the zeal of a Chinese shadow warrior. Weight loss at a sniff—what could be easier?

5. Ice Cube Diet

Yes, the main premise behind this celebrity weight loss diet is eating ice cubes. Made popular by a famous Hollywood actress, snacking on ice cubes apparently keeps hunger pangs at bay. Ice cubes as a snack… I must have missed their reclassification as a food item. Probably right around the time when the "Stupidest Fad Diets of the World," convention was happening. You guessed right. The main premise behind this celebrity weight loss diet is eating ice cubes. Made popular by a famous Hollywood actress, snacking on ice cubes apparently keeps hunger pangs at bay! So…ice cubes are a snack, huh? When did they get initiated into the food category? Right around the time when the "Stupidest Fad Diets of the World" convention was happening, I guess.

6. Cabbage Soup Diet

No doubt inspired by the Buckett family from Roald Dahl's Charlie and the Chocolate Factory, the Cabbage Soup diet has been one 34-year-old actress's lifeline when she needs to lose weight really, really fast. I can see why it works; I doubt anyone is going to go back for seconds. I guess that's how people following the cabbage soup diet stay in shape—they'd rather die than have any more!

As you can see, most of these celebrity weight loss diets border on the insane. They can't be sustained over a long period of time, and they certainly aren't the healthiest way to achieve weight loss. Rather than fall for these ridiculous, dangerous weight loss methods, it's best to adopt a holistic routine combining exercise, diet modification, and lifestyle changes, so you can lose weight and keep it off, without sacrificing your health in the process.

39

5 Simple, Practical and Effective Steps to Lose Your Face Fat and Get a Sculpted Face

If you're looking to lose face fat, the first thing you should consider is your lifestyle. No form of weight loss is possible or sustainable without a healthy lifestyle. There are no miracle diets or pills or facial exercises to lose face fat that will work magic in days. Unless you're willing to commit to the necessary lifestyle adjustments, you'll only end up frustrated.

1. Stress Is Your Enemy

The connection between facial fat and stress may seem flimsy at first, but controlling stress is one of the most crucial tips for losing facial fat. When you're stressed about something, the first thing it affects is the quality of your sleep. With improper sleep, your body becomes lethargic, and your metabolism slows down. A slow metabolism is the main cause of weight gain everywhere, including your face. Stress can also lead to bingeing on comfort food, and hormonal imbalances which lead to premature facial aging, such as loose, saggy skin.

2. Ways to Control Stress and Lose Facial Fat

Regular exercise is a great way to keep stress at bay. Also, try to keep yourself and your environment as calm and relaxed as possible at bedtime. Practicing meditation and yoga has helped many people deal with stress and insomnia.

3. The Problem of an Erratic Lifestyle

An erratic lifestyle can also be a major cause of weight gain, a puffy face, and fatigue. With your busy lifestyle, you probably have irregular eating and sleeping habits. That means your body is constantly confused; it never knows when to prepare to sleep, eat, or be active. Add excessive weekend drinking and a diet of fast food, and you have a recipe for disaster; poor diet and drinking will lead to weight gain, and fatigue to a sluggish metabolism.

The only way to perk up your metabolism and diet and lose the puffiness in your face is to practice routine and discipline. Maintain consistent sleeping hours, and actively control your drinking and dependence on high-calorie meals. Go for small drinks and low-calorie cocktails, if you must, and carry light, healthy snacks such as fruits, nuts or even whole-wheat sandwiches.

4. Smoking

Apart from all its other adverse effects, smoking deprives your body of vitamin C, which plays a big part in keeping your skin looking young and healthy. This leads to dull, sagging skin, which exaggerates your facial fat, making you look much older than your years.

5. The Need for Regular Exercise

Finally, if you *really* want to lose facial fat, or fat from anywhere else in your body, there's no substitute for regular exercise. Burning more calories than you consume is ultimately what causes weight loss, and the best way to achieve a calorie deficit is exercise. If you're pressed for time, try incorporating exercise into your regular routine, by taking walks on your breaks and the stairs instead of the elevator. If you incorporate these basic lifestyle adjustments, you should see a remarkable difference in just a few weeks.

40

How to Read Food Labels for Weight Loss

A healthy, low-calorie diet is essential for weight loss. But in a world which offers a million food choices, how can you control your diet? The answer is simple: by learning to read the nutritional label printed on packaged food.

A recent study conducted by Washington State University confirmed the value of this information. The study found that people who simply read food labels were more likely to lose weight than those who exercised, but ignored the labels. This is a significant finding; it shows that when you know how to read the nutritional information, you're better equipped to control the quantity of calories you consume in a day, and the quality of what you eat, resulting in a healthier diet and weight loss.

Serving Size

This is the first and most important piece of information the nutritional information label gives you; it suggests the amount of the given food you should consume in a serving. For instance, if you get a box of toaster pastries, the label says "Serving Size: 1 pastry." This means one pastry is all you should consume at one time. The serving size is calculated based on an average person's daily dietary requirement, or 2,000 calories. If you know your daily requirement based on your height and weight (and there are many calculators out there to help you determine this information, if you don't already know it), and your body requires 3,000 calories a day, the maximum serving size for you would be one-and-a-half times the recommended amount.

Number of Calories

Right next to the serving size, the label tells you the number of calories per serving. By paying attention to food labels, you'll be able to calculate the number of calories you consume in a day or week, and measure whether it's helping or hindering your weight loss efforts. Without this calorie information, you'll have a hard time measuring your diet. Typically, food items containing 200 or more calories per serving should be avoided for weight loss (unless, of course, a single serving is considered the nutritional equivalent of a full meal).

Information about Nutrients

Contrary to popular belief, counting calories isn't the only essential information for weight loss and good health. It's equally important to pay attention to the *quality* of what you're eating, and you can learn this from food labels as well. The nutritional information lists all the components of that food, including proteins, carbohydrates, fats, and nutrients.

Percent Daily Value

Additionally, the food label gives you the daily percentage of the nutrients in comparison to what you should be eating in total on a given day. For example, if a food item contains 7 grams of fat (the equivalent of 63 calories), it will show you the amount and then 10% in brackets. So this food contains 10% of the daily amount of fat you should be eating. Remember, this is based on a 2,000 calorie diet, so if your daily nutritional needs are different, you'll need to adjust these numbers accordingly.

The next time you shop, make sure you pay attention to the fine print and read the food labels carefully. Knowing serving size, calories, and nutritional quality will help you make more informed choices for better health and weight loss.

41

4 Ayurvedic Tips for Weight Loss

Many people dealing with the pressures of urban living struggle to successfully incorporate weight loss goals into their lives. Stress, irregular eating habits, poor sleep, and lack of exercise can all throw your body's systems completely out of balance, leading to health ills such as weight gain. In this context, the ancient system of Ayurveda is extremely relevant, because of its emphasis on the balance of energies in the human body. Following some simple Ayurvedic tips can help you vastly improve the quality of your life and health.

1. Regular Eating Habits

Your body's metabolism requires regularity. It needs to know what time to expect food, and the quantity and quality of the food it's about to receive. When you skip one or two meals a day, your body doesn't know when to expect its next meal, and when you do eat, it's caught unawares. As a result, your body stops metabolizing food efficiently, and fat reserves begin accumulating.

2. Eating the Right Things

Apart from regular eating habits, *what* you eat is also very important in order to lose weight with Ayurveda. Ayurveda recommends a Sattvic diet, a healthy and wholesome vegetarian diet with an emphasis on whole grains, nuts, lentils, fresh salads, cooked vegetables, a balance of herbs and spices, and fresh, seasonal fruits. You should never eat more food at any given time than you can hold in your cupped palms, or eat until you feel full and heavy. You should get up from a meal feeling light and energized.

3. Regular Exercise

Exercise is also crucial if you want to lose weight with Ayurveda; however, the same kind of exercise isn't beneficial for everyone. The type and volume of exercise you do should be based on your tendencies, and the unique balance of energies, or *doshas*, in your body.

4. Good Sleep

Above all, Ayurveda emphasizes that one thing is crucial for the physical and mental health of every individual—adequate sleep. Modern research backs this up, having linked poor sleep to several lifestyle ills, such as depression, stress, and poor metabolism. All of these, incidentally, lead to weight gain.

Though Ayurveda might be viewed as an "alternative" practice, it's evident in these tips for weight loss that there is a rational, scientific basis behind them, which should help anyone achieve their weight loss goals.

42

Summer Thirst Quenchers for Your Weight Loss Diet

It's certainly not advisable to stick to the same weight-loss plan year-round. Your diet should vary according to the needs and challenges of each season. In summer, the biggest challenge is keeping yourself hydrated. Temptation strikes several times a day, in the form of a cool, refreshing drink. Unfortunately, many of those drinks aren't compatible with weight loss. Here are a few tips to help you stick to your diet and quench your thirst.

Drinks to Avoid

Sodas count as among the unhealthiest summer drinks. A chilled soda might make you feel refreshed, but it's packed with sugar, calories, and harmful chemicals. Not only do they interfere with your weight loss goals, but sodas don't even hydrate your body. The sugar and caffeine they contain will make you feel thirsty again very quickly.

Most other cold drinks you find in cafes and stores, including iced teas, granitas, lemonades, juices and mocktails, all make the list of drinks to avoid, primarily because of the amount of sugar (and, consequently, calories) they contain. These are "empty" calories—they contain no nutritional value, aren't filling, and end up as excess pounds.

Homemade Substitutes

If you simply can't do without a flavorful, refreshing drink, try making your own lemonade or iced tea at home. If you can, make do with less or no sugar, or try a healthy sugar substitute such as unsweetened applesauce or pure maple syrup. You could try unsweetened green tea or fresh coconut water, too, for a thirst quencher with flavor. Coconut water also makes an excellent sports drink alternative; it contains high levels of balanced electrolytes to replenish your body after exercising in the heat.

Water

Water is the only liquid that has no calories and serves the sole purpose of hydrating your body, which makes it the most crucial summer thirst quencher, for weight loss or otherwise. If you deprive your body of water, the resulting dehydration will slow your metabolism, leading to a dip in energy levels and calorie burn. For your overall health and for weight loss, water needs to be your go-to drink. The one exception is if you're going to be working or playing sports outside in the heat; then you should make sure to drink 300–500 mL of a sports or electrolyte replacement drink. Just be careful; many sports drinks are loaded with sugar, so try diluting it with plain water, or, as suggested above, drink coconut water.

Fresh Fruit

This list is about beverages; why are we talking about fruit? Because the main component of fruit is water. Watermelon, for instance, lives up to its name at 95% water. Mangoes, melons and berries are all rich in water, too, and can help you stay hydrated. Most fruits contain essential electrolytes, too, which are crucial during summer.

Smoothies and Juices

Most fruit juices, smoothies, and mocktails aren't compatible with a weight loss diet. Fruit juice has none of the filling fiber of fruit, and fruit sugars only add empty calories to your system. Commercial smoothies and mocktails are often calorie bombs, and can contain 500 or more calories per glass, depending on the ingredients! If you must have a smoothie, make your own using whole fruits, low-fat yogurt, skim milk and ice.

While this list might not have contained any revelations, it's a good reminder of the principles.

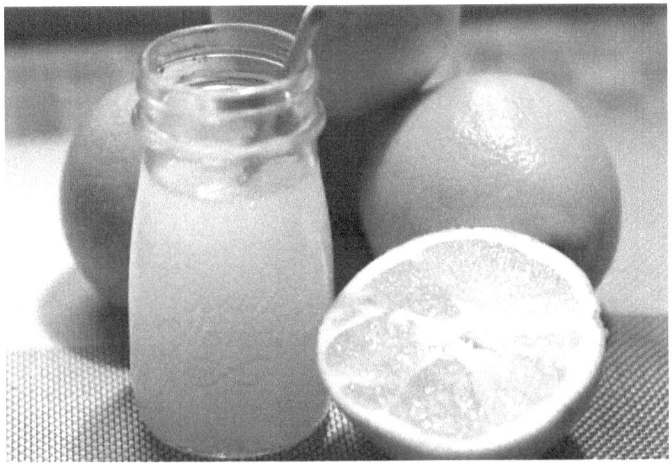

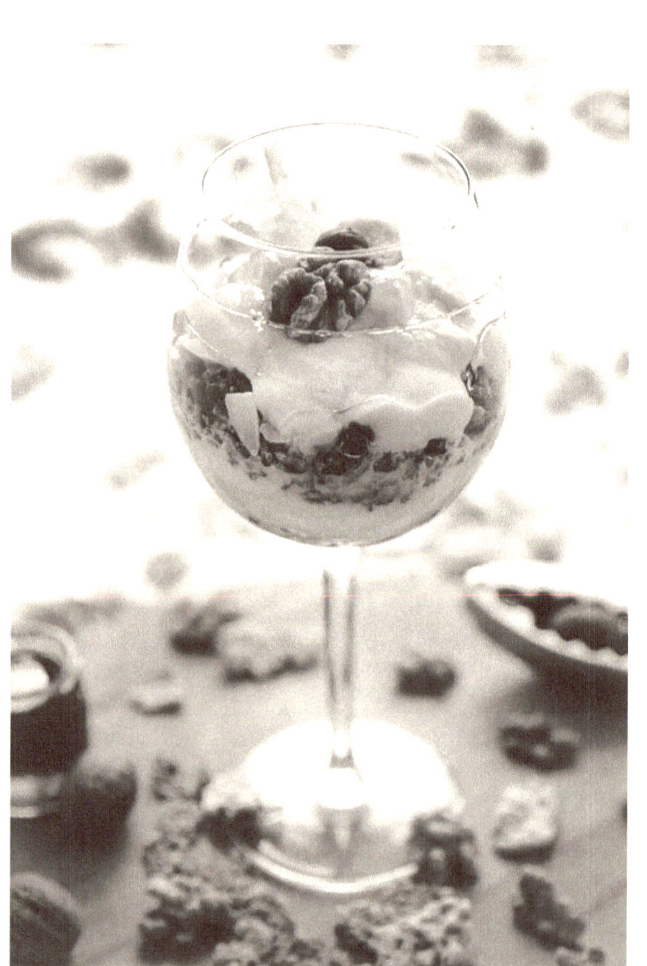

43

How to Succeed with a Summer Weight Loss Diet

You may be aiming to lose weight this season or even this year, but summer has the power to break your resolve. It's the season of vacations, beach holidays and parties. Amid all the revelries, it's easy to forget yourself and indulge, and before you know it, you've put on weight. It is possible to bypass this vicious cycle, though, and still have fun. Here are some tips for an effective summer diet plan.

Drink a Lot of Water

The biggest risk you face in summer is dehydration. When you're out having fun, it's easy to forget your body's simplest need: water. Even if you're not doing any strenuous physical activity, your body constantly loses water when it's hot, and if you don't replenish it, your metabolism slows with dehydration. Of course, when your metabolism slows, you burn fewer calories, and run a greater risk of putting on weight. You might even misinterpret thirst as hunger and overeat. So, to prevent disaster, keep water handy at all times, and keep sipping. It's one of the simplest and most essential aspects of weight loss.

Eat Fresh Fruit

Summer is the season for berries and tropical fruits, so take advantage! Fruit is nutritious, high in fiber and water content, to keep you full and hydrated, and are relatively low in calories. And fresh fruit is a lot healthier than fruit juice or a sweetened smoothie. You can even turn snacking into a fun family outing, by heading to a local orchard or berry farm to pick your own fruit.

Control your Portions

Give yourself some latitude—you're on vacation, after all—but enjoy food within limits. Portion control is the best way to have your cheesy lasagna and eat it too. Instead of wolfing down a plateful by yourself, share your dish with a friend or your partner.

Healthy Eating is Possible

Make sure that, with each meal, there's a healthy, low-calorie component. Instead of fries, have steamed veggies with your burger. Additionally, if you can make a commitment to have one meal a day that's completely healthy and low in calories, you'll have an excellent chance at summer weight loss success.

Don't Skip Meals

After overindulging, people tend to skip a meal out of guilt and a misguided attempt to undo the damage they've done. This won't help you lose or even control weight, though, especially if you do it on a regular basis. You'll only confuse your body, and it will respond with a sluggish metabolism and low energy levels—exactly what you want to avoid on vacation. The success of your summer diet will also depend heavily on how well you control your intake of alcohol. Alcohol is high in calories on its own; cocktails are veritable calorie bombs. So, sip your drink slowly, and stick to no more than one or two small drinks in an evening, once a week.

These tips will easily save you 500–600 calories a day, and it adds up quickly; by the end of the summer, you could be looking at a new you!

44

How to Lose 9 Pounds Fast: How about Weight Loss Supplements?

Many people who lead metropolitan lifestyles around the world end up overweight or even obese. As a result, there are millions of people out there desperately trying to find a way to lose nine pounds fast. This is why the weight loss product industry has become a multi-billion dollar giant. Weight loss supplements, in particular, offer the ultimate temptation: pop a magic pill, and start losing weight fast. The method appeals to our age and attitudes—but how effective is it really?

How Dramatic Are the Results?

If you want to lose nine pounds fast by using diet supplements, you have to understand the full implications. There are dozens of weight loss supplements out there promising dramatic results, but the simple fact is that no supplement has yet been manufactured which is an effective weight loss solution by itself. All these supplements claim to either increase metabolism, suppress appetites, or block fat absorption, but none of them will really work unless you adopt an exercise regime and a healthy diet. Even the most effective supplements will, at best, marginally enhance the results of an already healthy diet plan. If you think a weight loss supplement is going to boost your metabolism without the crucial support of a healthy diet, you're on the wrong track.

The Side Effects

One thing that concerns people—and rightly so—is the side effects of weight loss supplements. In an alarming study conducted by the Food and Drug

Administration (FDA) of the U.S. recently, it was found that dozens of so-called "herbal" supplements are using lab-produced prescription drugs and ingredients in their pills and products, in a bid to come up with a more effective weight loss formula. The dosages of some of these ingredients were reported to be much higher than recommended, and could cause side effects and dangerous medication interactions for people taking other medicines. Consumers are also being given incomplete information on the labels of the products they're purchasing, believing them to be completely natural and safe. Thermogenic supplements, as well as natural herbs and extracts like Hoodia Godonii and Bitter Orange, are all under fire for the damage they can potentially cause to a body's vital organs and processes, especially the liver and heart. So don't feel safe with a supplement, just because it claims to be herbal. The FDA itself recommends that people should only trust a product or brand after consulting a qualified physician.

The Verdict

All the supposed benefits of weight loss supplements are not the product of some magic formula. You can achieve the same results by following a healthy lifestyle and exercising 2–3 hours a week. Your choices aren't limited to sweating it out in a gym ten hours a week or popping a pill. There's a healthy middle ground even the busiest person can find time for. And, considering the potentially damaging side effects of weight loss supplements, the dubious information and misinformation available about them, and their largely unimpressive real-world results, they're best avoided. Try, instead, a truly natural weight to lose weight quickly and easily—it works!

45

How to Make Your Weight Loss Plan a Success!

Just like every other year, more than 80% of people will fail in their plan to lose weight this year. In my experience as a fitness professional, I've encountered dozens of people who start off with the ambition to lose weight quickly. Sadly, most of them jump ship within the first month. If you don't want to be one of them, read on and find out just how you can successfully follow through with your weight loss plan this year.

Emotional Decision Making

When people realize they're overweight, they usually feel a combination of panic, guilt, and anger. In their emotionally charged state, they jump into an ambitious weight loss plan with both feet. "I'll give up sweets," "I won't have more than one drink a week," "I'll go to the gym for an hour and a half every day." The result of that emotional decision making is frustration and failure. The faces change every year, but it's the same story, with the same result. What they don't understand is that goals should only be set when you're thinking clearly, and those goals should be broken down into gradual, practical steps.

The Miracle of Small Changes

I want you to be the exception, to understand that losing weight quickly doesn't require drastic steps. If you can make gradual and sustainable changes in your life, you'll succeed. Here's an example: Say you weigh 190 pounds, and are consuming a maintenance level of calories (an amount which will cause you to neither lose nor gain weight). If you can make just one small change in your lifestyle, like adding twenty minutes of exercise a day, or swapping your afternoon can of soda for a piece of fruit, you'll end up burning about 200 calories more than you consume every day, on average. With just one small change, you'll end up burning 6,000 calories more than you consume in a month. In a year, that will lead to a weight loss of twenty pounds! By the time the New Year rolls around, your weight loss plan will have succeeded. And if you don't lose any weight, that means if you'd continued with your habits, you would have *gained* twenty pounds. However you look at it, every small change has the potential to make a big difference to your weight loss plan. The only caveat is that it must be *sustainable* change.

If you're serious about losing weight quickly, start by omitting some of the junk food you eat every day, and replace it with wholesome, nutritious foods. You don't have to give up sweets completely; change, in any amount, if sustained over time, will make a difference. The same goes for exercise. If you find something you like and can stick with it, you'll see results. Be patient, monitor your progress, and craft your weight loss plan in a calm, rational frame of mind. If you can do that, you're already on your way to success!

46

Celebrity Weight Loss Diets: The Kind You Should Never Follow

Everyone, celebrities included, wants to lose weight fast. We're not alone in our desire to get a slim body as fast as possible. Living in a generation that's pressed for time from every possible angle, instant answers and quick solutions are very, very tempting.

But how reliable are these fad diets? They might offer *rapid* weight loss, but is it *healthy?* Most people are so desperate, they don't care about the consequences so much as the results of following these diets. The appeal increases tenfold when we see our favorite celebrities, sleek and svelte, endorsing—either directly or indirectly—the drastic measures which helped them achieve their picture-perfect figure.

One of the more popular celebrity diet plans is Master Cleanse—a diet which only allows you to drink a concoction of lemon juice, maple syrup, cayenne pepper, and water. One Hollywood celebrity lost twenty pounds in two weeks while following the Master Cleanse, but who wouldn't, if they were surviving on little more than water. And the singer confessed that she gained the weight back as soon as the diet was over.

One famous actress swears by the Cabbage Soup diet, while another two endorse the baby food diet. A supermodel credits her figure to the Raw Food diet, while a famous socialite/model's secret is the Cookie Diet.

At some point, you have to stop and ask the question, "How healthy are these diets?" The main strategy of fad diets is to severely restrict the number of calories you consume, generally leading to accelerated weight loss. That's the *only* advantage (if you can call it that) of following such a drastic, limited diet.

On the other hand, the list of the disadvantages of these insane techniques is a mile long. First, the rapid weight loss they achieve is unsafe and unsustainable. According to the Mayo Clinic, you should lose no more than one or two pounds per week during safe, sustainable weight loss. Anything more than that is a potential health risk—it can lead to lean muscle, tissue, and even bone density loss. These diets also fall far short when it comes to providing your body with the basic, essential nutrition it needs to perform day-to-day functions.

The temptation of rapid, nearly effortless weight loss is strong, but personally, I prefer losing weight loss in the long term. I don't want to starve myself, restrict the kinds of food I eat, and deny myself wholesome meals, so I can be slender for a few days before packing the pounds back on. I'd rather lose weight slowly while feeling strong, healthy and satisfied, and keep it off, thanks to the sustainable changes I've made. Hopefully, you'll make the choice to improve your health as well as your waistline, too.

47

The Best Foods to Burn Fat

I f you've set out to lose weight, you probably know that diet, as well as exercise, is going to be a crucial part of your plan. The problem is that most easily available, ready-made foods aren't conducive to exercise and weight loss. So, it's important to learn which foods are the best to help burn fat, and stock up accordingly. Bear in mind these foods are suggested under the assumption that you're following some sort of exercise plan to lose weight.

Oatmeal

If you're exercising regularly, healthy carbohydrates are the most critical part of your diet. Your body turns carbs into glucose, the fuel which powers your muscles. Oatmeal is a rich source of healthy complex carbohydrates, which is why it appears near the top of every list of healthy foods for exercise and weight loss. Complex carbohydrates are digested slowly, providing a sustained release of sugar in your bloodstream. This keeps you energized through your workout, and even after, helping to curb post-exercise munchies. Whole, unprocessed oats, such as steel-cut, are the best form of oatmeal for weight loss, as they keep you fuller longer, making you less likely to overeat.

Coffee

If you love your coffee, don't feel guilty—it loves you, too! As long as you're not overindulging, coffee is an excellent addition to a diet and exercise plan. Drink twelve ounces an hour or so before your workout, and it can help boost your endurance. Coffee also eases post-workout muscular fatigue and soreness, helping you last longer and recover faster. Your workouts will be more productive, and you'll have a better chance of achieving your weight loss goals. Coffee can be dehydrating, but if consumed in moderation, you shouldn't have a problem.

Almonds and Raisins

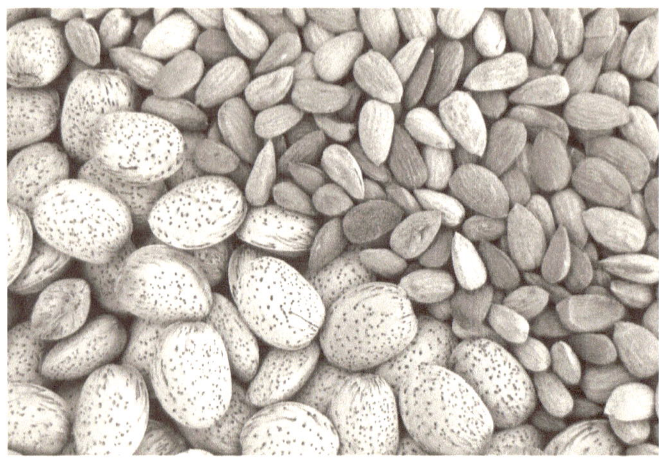

Dry fruits and nuts are healthy snacks, and almonds and raisins particularly so, especially in conjunction with an exercise plan. Almonds are rich in antioxidants, which counter the harmful free radicals produced by your body during intense exercise, and they also boost endurance.

Raisins are packed with more energy than any commercially-produced energy bar. They're full of potassium, which can prevent dehydration after a workout, and are loaded with vital carbohydrates as well.

Water and Tomato Juice

If you work out for less than an hour, and it's not severely hot or humid, you don't need a sports drink. Plain water is your most crucial necessity, so fill up your bottle at home and pick up a banana or two instead of a sugary sports drink. If you do work out for more than an hour and you've sweated profusely, you need to replace not just the water you've lost, but also vital electrolytes such as potassium and sodium. Dilute a glass of pure tomato juice, and you've got an excellent electrolyte replacement drink. One glass of tomato juice contains six to fifteen times more potassium and sodium than a regular sports drink.

48

Choosing Healthy Office Snacks for Weight Loss

The challenge of a busy work life and attempting to lose weight simultaneously may seem daunting. Even if you can't take time out for exercise, though, there's no reason you can't choose healthy office snacks for when those late-afternoon hunger pangs strike. Instead of reaching for the candy bowl or a fast-food burger, try these healthy foods instead.

Fruit

If you want something tasty, healthy, light and filling, there's no better choice than seasonal fruit. Keep two or three different types handy, so you have variety in taste and nutrition. Make sure the fruits you choose are easy to carry and munch on. Grapes, apples, bananas, pears and berries all fit the bill. If your office has a full kitchen and you're in the mood for something more filling, you could whip up a fresh banana shake or smoothie, with low-fat milk and yogurt. And healthy breakfast cereal with added fresh fruit makes a delicious, refreshing light meal.

Nuts

Nuts are essential to any diet. They're an excellent source of muscle-building protein, they battle hunger pangs, and also contain essential healthy fats. They are rich in calories, though, so make sure your portion is no bigger than an ounce. That still gives you roughly 25 almonds! Just avoid the salted varieties, and have the plain roasted ones instead. And just like fruit, nuts make a great addition to a healthy low-fat shake or breakfast cereal.

Peanut Butter and Whole Wheat Crackers

Whole-wheat and multi-grain crackers are fiber-rich and unrefined. Add a dab of peanut butter, and you have a tasty, protein-rich, wholesome snack that'll keep you fuller longer. Just pay attention to portion sizes, particularly in regards to the peanut butter.

Instant Oatmeal

Instant oatmeal is nutritious, light in calories (110 calories per serving) and filling. All you need to do is heat and eat. If you want to enhance the flavor, add cinnamon, raisins or chopped fruit. Oatmeal's combination of nutrition, convenience, and versatility make it one of the best office snacks for weight loss.

Snack Bars

If you're looking to lose weight, make sure to read the nutritional information carefully. Avoid high-calorie bars loaded with sugar, which are really little better than candy bars. Choose ones with a small and natural list of ingredients, with little or no added sugar, under 200 calories per serving. The best snack bars contain whole-grain ingredients, nuts, and dried fruit.

Of course, all these snacks require some prior planning. If you only start thinking about what to eat when hunger pangs strike, you'll reach for whatever is closest. That's why, if you're serious about losing weight, you need to keep healthy snacks readily available. As you can see from this list, once you've stocked up, there's little to no preparation required. These foods will also keep you energized through the day, and you'll feel more confident about your weight loss goals.

49

The Value of a Healthy Breakfast for Weight Loss

How important is a healthy breakfast? Despite being one of the most commonly asked questions on the subject of health and weight loss, there's no ambiguity to the answer—a healthy breakfast is crucial to your diet.

A Light Breakfast is Fine

Contrary to popular belief, you don't have to fill up with a full country breakfast early in the day. If you don't wake up hungry, that's fine. You can begin your day with something light, and wait a few hours before beginning your eating cycle. But if you're trying to follow a diet for weight loss, it's crucial that whatever you have in the morning is nutritious.

The Problem with Sugar-Rich Foods

If you fill up with sugar-rich foods in the morning, you'll be loading up on calories and 'quick-release' carbohydrates. These carbs are digested rapidly, and in spite of the number of calories you've consumed, you'll end up feeling hungry again very soon. The rush of sugar in your blood will crash rapidly, too, leaving you starving and exhausted well before lunchtime.

Traditional Choices to Knock off Your List

For this reason, many traditional breakfast foods should be ruled out: sugary breakfast cereals, pastries, muffins, pancakes, waffles, donuts, pies and scones. Other items, like fried eggs and sausage, cheesy omelets, cream cheese covered bagels, and hash browns, are fatty, greasy calorie bombs.

The Right Ingredients

A healthy breakfast should consist of protein, fiber, and complex carbohydrates. Each of these ingredients will keep you feeling fuller longer, and release energy to your bloodstream slowly and steadily, leaving you feeling energetic and bright, without the urge to overeat.

Eggs

Eggs, specifically egg whites, are rich in protein, an essential part of a healthy diet. The best way to have your eggs is boiled or poached, but for more taste, you could scramble them in olive oil and add vegetables such as onions, peppers and tomatoes. Toasted whole wheat bread with low-fat butter makes an excellent side dish.

Whole Grains

Whole grains offer the right kind of carbohydrates and are rich in fiber, which is why whole wheat cereal is also recommended. If you like cereal, a bowl of oatmeal might appeal to you, and it's the best choice for weight loss. Instead of adding sugar, try adding dried fruits and nuts, berries, or bananas, for a tasty, wholesome, and filling breakfast to keep you energized until lunch.

Light Bites

If you prefer something lighter, try low-fat yogurt with fresh fruit, or even a fruit salad. You can also try blending whole fruits like berries or bananas with low-fat yogurt or milk, for a tasty, homemade smoothie.

50

The Gym for Weight Loss: 5 Essential Tips

Many people find working out in a gym helps them stay disciplined and motivated toward achieving their weight loss goals. The availability of a professional fitness trainer to help you learn the correct way to perform the exercises provides an edge to your workout routine, too. So, if you're planning to join a gym to lose weight fast, here's some essential information.

The Gym is Not Indispensable for Weight Loss

While you may be looking forward to joining a gym, understand that it's not a mandatory component of a weight loss routine. Countless people have succeeded at weight loss without joining a gym, simply by implementing a personal exercise plan and a balanced, healthy diet. Even if you don't have the time or money to sign up with a gym just yet, you can still start losing weight.

A Good Trainer

If you've never worked out in a gym before, you might feel lost the first time you walk in. That's why it's imperative to seek the guidance of a trained fitness instructor. Any good trainer will learn about your physical capabilities, objectives, and exercise and medical history, before getting you started. If a trainer tries to start you on a plan without collecting this information first, that's a red flag; steer clear.

Acclimatizing

As far as muscle-building and strengthening is concerned, you need to start slowly and focus on learning the right form and posture, before challenging yourself with heavier weights or more repetitions. For the first few weeks, your body will still be getting used to this new demand—don't overstrain yourself and cripple your fitness efforts.

Cardiovascular Exercises

If your objective is to lose weight, you'll need to focus on cardiovascular exercises, such as walking, running, rowing or cycling. A gym has several different types of equipment for cardiovascular exercises, and each of these offers your body a different kind of challenge. There's the stationary bike, the elliptical cross trainer, the treadmill, and the rowing machine. All of these offer different types of cardio workouts for your individual needs. For instance, if you've suffered an impact-related injury to one of your legs from excessive walking or running, it's best to stick to the stationary bike, rowing machine, or even the elliptical. If you have trouble with your back, your best fit might be the recumbent bike.

Warm Up and Cool Down

It's also very important to do a proper warm-up and cooldown at the beginning and end of your session. Beginners often forget this, but the stretching at the beginning of your workout keeps your body supple and prevents workout injuries and strains. A cooldown helps flush your muscles of built-up lactic acid which causes soreness, aiding your recovery.

Rest and Recovery

Finally, make sure to give yourself enough rest and recovery time. It's only in the period of rest following your workout that your muscles grow and adapt, making you stronger. As a beginner, you shouldn't be visiting the gym more than four or five times a week.

51

The Fascinating Weight Loss Story of Adam Reitz

Many people begin the season with weight loss and fitness goals, and most are on the hunt for exciting, fail-proof methods to lose weight. Adam Reitz, a school teacher from Bethlehem, Pennsylvania, is a worthy inspiration to all such people. He's shown how one can successfully and sustainably lose even 100 pounds, using the most ancient and simple form of exercise: running. Here's an account of how to lose weight, the Adam Reitz way.

The Inspiration

Just before his wedding three years ago, Adam Reitz weighed a whopping 275 pounds. His fiancee, also a teacher at the same school, accompanied him on a class trip. When Adam saw the photos of the trip, all he could see was a fat man standing next to his future wife. He'd been aware of his weight before, but it had never really hit him until that moment. He was profoundly disgusted with himself, but rather than wallow in self-pity, his negative feelings spurred him into action. With his wedding coming up, Adam was determined to make changes. He didn't sign up for any fad diets; he just eliminated junk food, controlled his diet, and started riding his bicycle. By the time his wedding rolled around, he'd shed twenty pounds, which earned him a lot of compliments and motivated him still further.

Addicted to Running

At this stage, Adam's friend convinced him to sign up for a half-marathon, and that's where his love affair with running started. He couldn't even run one block when he began, but slowly, he became addicted to the challenge and thrill of running. Gradually, he began to feel healthier, fitter, and leaner.

In 2008, he participated in the Philadelphia marathon, by which time he'd lost 50 pounds. He went on to do a marathon in Washington in under four hours, and finally, the New York City Marathon. For this one, he prepared intensively, dedicating his Saturdays to training. He and his friends did a 20 mile run every other week, and on the day of the race, Adam reached the finish line in under 3 ½ hours, an elite time. By now, this once-obese man had reached his ideal weight of 175 pounds, and his size 44 waist had shrunk to a 32, in just three years. It was a remarkable change.

The Lessons

The most striking feature of Adam's journey is how he did it. He didn't go on a starvation diet, or rush out to purchase diet pills, or sign up for bizarre methods. He made healthy, sustainable lifestyle changes, and his objectives were to lose weight as well as get healthier. Everyone who wants to lose weight can draw inspiration from Adam's example. You don't have to start running marathons; losing weight doesn't always require extreme lifestyle changes. Simply committing to regulating your diet and incorporating exercise is enough.

52

4 Healthy Habits for Fast Weight Loss in a Matter of Days

If you want to lose weight fast, stop looking for secrets, magic tricks, or wonder pills. Fitness and nutrition experts have been telling us the answer for years—in order to lose weight, you need to adopt healthy habits. Whether you want to lose ten pounds or fifty, it's not just about getting slim, but staying slim. That's not going to happen, unless you start living healthy.

Fruits and Veggies

In order to get slim, you need to get natural, which means incorporating more fruits and vegetables into your diet. Fresh veggies and fruits are rich in complex carbohydrates and nutrients, and fiber, and they're low in calories. With all the fiber in a full serving of fruits or veggies, you'll be left feeling fuller longer, and will be less tempted to overeat. Your calorie count comes down, and you're on the right track for weight loss.

Try adding an extra portion of fruits or veggies to your favorite meals, like breakfast cereal, pasta, or casseroles. You can also add a side of steamed vegetables with dinner, or a fresh fruit salad for dessert.

Get Moving

Literally. Moving is what you need to do in order to lose weight fast. Whether you want to go cycling with friends, use your bike to commute, or incorporate a brisk walk into your routine, some form of cardiovascular exercise is crucial to slim down. With a healthier diet, you'll be able to cut calories and improve your metabolism a bit, but for fast weight loss, you need a serious jump in the calories you're burning per day, and that can only come from exercise. If nothing else, simply adding more activity into your daily life counts, like taking the stairs, parking your car farther away from your destination, and walking for errands.

Eliminate Junk

Eliminating addictive processed foods is easier said than done, but it's a necessary step, if you're serious about changing your diet for weight loss. Don't try to go cold turkey; such rapid, sudden switches are hard to sustain. Instead, try reducing your portions of processed food, and replace them with a more wholesome food choice. So, if tomorrow's lunch is a burger, replace the soda with a homemade banana smoothie.

Get Stronger

You know by now that muscle burns more calories than fat. The more lean muscle you acquire, the faster your metabolism will be, and the quicker you'll get slim. Try to incorporate two 15–30 minute sessions of strength training into your routine every week. Once your muscles are toned, your body shape will improve, too, and you'll feel stronger, sexier, and more energetic.

You don't have to complete these toning sessions in a gym. There are plenty of strength exercises you can do in your living room, using your own body weight (squats, leg raises, push-ups, chair dips, etc). If you feel you need a bit more guidance, there are plenty of exercise videos and even apps out there you can follow along with.

53

5 Steps to Lose Weight Permanently

If you're frustrated by constant failed efforts at losing weight, and the yo-yoing numbers on the scale, perhaps it's time to sit back for a moment. I guarantee you haven't been consistently following at least two or more of the five crucial weight loss steps described below. Once you understand and commit to following them, you'll finally be on a path for successful, permanent weight loss.

Step 1: Stop Seeking Short Cuts

Of course, if you go on a fancy diet plan which strictly regulates every meal and drastically cuts your carbohydrate consumption, you're going to lose weight. However, it'll also slow your metabolism, make you tired and lethargic, and can even cause nutritional imbalances. The worst thing is that it's a wasted effort; as soon as you return to your normal eating habits, that extra weight will return to you. So stop looking for a magic pill, diet, or drink. There are no short cuts to weight loss, and no substitutes for a disciplined approach and proper plan.

Step 2: Stop Drifting and Set a Goal!

Speaking of planning, don't be one of the many people who proclaim they want to lose weight, but have no specific goals in place to do it. Usually, this sort of half-hearted effort only lasts for a few days. What you need is a target, like losing twelve pounds by summer. Now divide that target into achievable, short-term weight loss goals. How about losing a pound in the first ten days? In order to do that, you'll need to burn about 300 calories more than you consume in a day.

Step 3: Pick Up a Sport or a Fun Exercise

Are you one of those people who thinks there's no place but a gym for fitness? Now's the time to broaden your horizons. Your body doesn't care where it is; it burns calories just as efficiently on the road, the soccer field, or even in your living room. You're better off finding something fun and enjoyable, like a sport, jogging, or bicycling, than you are toiling away in a gym five days a week, especially if you're new to fitness. You'll actually look forward to your workout, burn a lot of calories, and later, if you want, you can always build on it.

Step 4: Discard The Junk, But Slowly...

Alcohol, sweets, burgers, fries, sundaes…you already know these things will disrupt your weight loss goals. If you go cold-turkey and swear never to touch a sweet again, though, you're setting yourself up for stress and frustration. Successful weight loss is all about moderation. Even if you cut your consumption of problem foods in half, you'll have made a *big* change. So, if you have a burger five days a week, cut that down to two days, to begin with. Then, once you've acclimated to eating healthier, you can make burgers an occasional treat. Lots of successful dieters allow themselves a "cheat" meal every week, as a reward for sticking to a healthy diet the rest of the time.

Step 5: Bring In Healthy Food

If you're not eating junk food, what are you supposed to survive on? Healthy food, of course, especially if you want to lose weight fast. Stock your fridge and pantry with fruits, veggies, wholesome meals, lots of water, and lean proteins like low-fat milk products, egg whites, beans, whole grains, and lean meats.

54

How to Lose 10 Pounds Fast – 4 New Tips for Fast and Amazing Results

When people begin the year with a fitness target such as losing ten pounds, they're not talking about six months from now; they want to lose it *fast*. While most health experts recommend gradual weight loss through sustainable changes, there are ways to fast-track the process without compromising your health. It'll take effort and discipline on your part, but your reward will be success, improved energy levels, and a killer physique.

1. Burn More and Consume Less

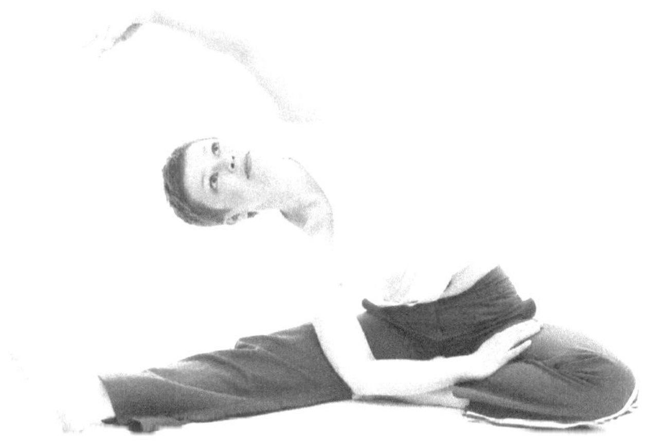

If you want to lose those ten pounds fast, you need to burn more calories than you consume to drop those extra pounds. The key word there is *burn*; restricting calories isn't the answer. Cutting your intake of food drastically will force your body into starvation mode, slowing your metabolism—not to mention you'll be miserable. Your energy levels will suffer, too, and as soon as you give up—as you inevitably will—those pounds will come back with interest. What you need to do is cut your calorie intake by a reasonable amount and boost your metabolism simultaneously. That's how you lose weight fast.

2. A Good Quality Diet

If you want to cut calories and boost your metabolism through your diet, you should emphasize not the *quantity* of your diet, but its *quality.* Not all calories are created equal. If you have a wholesome 400 calorie meal, the effects on your weight loss goals will be very different than if you have a 400 calorie bar of chocolate. First, your body's digestive system takes much longer to break down and process the healthy meal. The longer the digestive process, the more calories burned during the process. This slower digestive process also means your body is kept full and satisfied for longer, protecting you from the urge to overeat. On the other hand, the chocolate will be processed much more quickly, and since your body doesn't receive any significant nutrition, you'll be hungry again in no time and searching for a snack. If you really want to lose weight fast, the majority of your meals should be wholesome and nutritious. Avoid processed and junk foods as much as possible.

3. Eat Frequently

This might seem counterintuitive, but if you're going to consume 2,000 calories in a day, it's best to distribute that number over five or six meals, rather than two or three. The more times your body is required to burn calories, the faster your metabolism will be. And since your body can expect frequent meals, it won't feel obliged to store fat for a rainy day.

4. Regular Exercise

The other way to kick-start your metabolism is with regular exercise. If you can find time to spare every week for a sport or exercise, you'll burn more calories and have a better chance of losing weight quickly and achieving your overall goals.

55

Dance Your Way to Weight Loss Success – 5 Tips Revealed

It can be difficult to get excited about fitness. Setting out to an aerobics class, lugging yourself up on the treadmill, and lifting weights all sound like frightening, tiresome chores. If so, you don't need to be disheartened—the gym is not the only fitness solution available. What about having fun while losing weight? If that sounds ideal, dance might be just what you're looking for.

1. Calories Burned With Dancing

Any form of vigorous dancing is an excellent exercise for weight loss, because it burns a *lot* of calories. In one hour, you can burn anywhere in the range of 400–600 calories, depending on your body weight and the intensity of the dance. This is just as much, if not more, as you'd burn cycling, walking, or swimming. It's no wonder dancing is regarded as one of the best cardiovascular workouts available.

2. Ideal for Weight Loss

Experts agree that two-and-a-half hours of cardiovascular exercise a week is necessary for an average person to maintain fitness and a healthy body weight. Simply by going to a few classes a week, and practicing your moves at home now and then, you could lose 3–4 pounds a month, an ideal rate of weight loss. Obviously, this will only happen by maintaining a healthy diet in conjunction with dance.

3. The Most Effective Dance Forms

There are many forms of dance, so which ones burn the most calories? Belly dancing and energetic Latin dances come out on top. Rumba, samba, salsa, jive and cha-cha will all put you in a serious weight loss zone. Fast jazz-style dancing and hip-hop are just as effective, though hip-hop can be too acrobatic for those without a solid dance background. There are lots of dance classes available; it shouldn't be hard to find a style you enjoy.

4. Other Health Advantages

Dance isn't just a great weight loss exercise; it also keeps your cardiovascular system healthy and tones your muscles. Toned muscles boost your metabolic rate, which in turn burns more calories, even when you're at rest. It also improves flexibility, and can even improve bone density in women.

5. Growing Popularity

The best part is that dancing for exercise is becoming increasingly popular, so most gyms offer several classes to keep up with the demand. You'll likely find one in your neighborhood, and it probably won't be too expensive, either.

Apart from its health and weight loss benefits, learning a form of dance is a very enriching cultural experience, one that gives you a chance to make friends and connect with your body in a new way. So, what are you waiting for?

56

4 Weight Loss Foods to Avoid That Make You Put on Weight!

Several million people around the world are currently dieting, so the rapid rate at which the 'health food' industry is growing should come as no surprise. Everyone is trying to convince you that their product is fresh, wholesome, healthy, and rich in all sorts of nutrients. Don't be taken in by this proliferation of so-called weight loss foods. Here are some food items whose marketing can fool you into thinking they're healthy, but have the potential to derail your weight loss goals.

1. Smoothies

You'd probably never guess this one; after all, what could be wrong with a fruit-rich smoothie? First of all, most commercial smoothies are made with fruit *juice*, not whole fruit, so you get all of the sugar but none of the fiber. And the frozen yogurt or sherbet component loads the drink with sugar and calories. You might have a drink that satisfies like a light snack, but you've paid a full meal's worth of calories for it—as much as 600 calories. If you're really craving a smoothie, make one at home, with whole fruit and low-fat yogurt.

2. Granola

It's tasty, and it seems like it should be loaded with nutrients, but what it's really full of is calories. Most granola cereals have more sugar than fiber, too, so your body will be asking for seconds, even though you already ate 500 calories worth of cereal. When choosing breakfast cereal, find one that has more fiber than sugar, and add your own sweetness and flavor with fruit and nuts.

3. Salad

Salad is the first thing we think of in terms of diet food. And rightly so; a homemade salad is full of delicious and healthy greens, lean meat, egg white and beans. But the salads you buy in commercial outlets and restaurants have a lot of other ingredients that really pile on the calories, like cheese, bacon, and creamy dressings. Believe it or not, that bowl of salad could contain 1,000 calories—the same as a burger meal!

4. Energy Bars

Many people have already figured out this scam, but there are still a few unfortunate people buying into the supposed merits of energy bars. Most energy bars are similar to granola—packed with sugar and sweeteners, and low in fiber. Some are even rich in saturated fat. These 'light snacks' will give you a meal's worth of calories, and probably won't even hold you until lunch or dinner. If you must shop for an energy bar, read the label, and choose one with 200 or fewer calories per serving, and whole grain ingredients like whole oat, whole wheat, or brown rice. And, if possible, try to get one with at least 5 grams of protein, 3 grams of fiber, and less than 2 grams of saturated fat.

57

Make Your Weight Loss Workout at Home a Success

As serious as you are about wanting to lose weight fast, you simply might not be able to make it to the gym for your workouts. There are a number of potential obstacles, after all, like time, cost, or distance. You can work out at home, or course, but the question is, can you successfully do a weight loss workout at home? The simple answer is yes, you can. The challenge isn't in finding the right exercises—there are limitless options for working out at home, with or without equipment—but in finding motivation in a home environment.

Comfort as an Obstacle

The main reason people find it easy to work out in a gym is that there's simply not much else to do there; it's a place specifically designed for exercise. You're also likely to find motivation and inspiration in a gym environment, surrounded by so many other people sweating it out. While your home is a convenient and comfortable place for exercise, it's a little *too* comfortable, and many people struggle to establish focus.

Plan The Time

The biggest challenge of working out at home is the number of distractions. The phone rings, the kids interrupt, your spouse needs you to run an errand or fix something, and the television and computer are only a few steps away. The first thing you need to do is eliminate these distractions. Plan in advance for a certain time of the day, four to five times a week, just as you would if you were going to the gym, and stay disciplined. Once you're prepared, bring your family into the loop, so they know exactly when it is you're not to be disturbed.

Plan Your Workout

You'll also need to plan the type of workout you'll be doing. Keep in mind spacial restraints, available equipment, and time. There are tons of workouts you can do without any special equipment at all, so don't let that stop you. Even if the exercise video you're following calls for light hand weights, you can substitute soup cans or full water bottles.

Designate a Place

Once you've determined the content of your workout, you need to designate a space in your home to complete it. It should preferably be a place with as little distraction as possible, like a basement, attic, or spare bedroom. Try not to have things you associate with comfort within range, either; if there's a couch in the room, turn your back on it!

Beware of the Phone

Unless you're using a workout app, keep your phone out of reach during your workout, and keep a towel, water, a clock, and anything else you'll need close at hand. You don't want to stop midway through your exercises to run to the kitchen for some water; it's distracting, and it'll upset your rhythm.

58

Weight Loss Diet – How to Plan Low Calorie Dinner Recipes

You know a healthy, low-calorie dinner is a crucial part of dieting for weight loss. It's important to educate yourself, therefore, on what exactly constitutes a low-calorie dinner, and what foods you should avoid. Healthy weight loss isn't just a matter of calorie-counting—choosing the right things to eat and the right times of day to eat them is equally, if not more, important. If you're not eating the right things, you'll be unable to control your calorie intake, or improve your body's metabolism and energy levels.

Eat Light

The last thing you need is a carbohydrate kick at night; your body's processes are slowing down as it prepares for sleep. Respect that, and eat light. A heavy meal will both pile on the calories and affect the quality of your sleep; it's common knowledge that a full stomach is a formula for a restless night's sleep. If you don't get enough sleep, you cripple your metabolism still further, preventing your body from burning as many calories as you should.

The Best Food Items

Ideally, a low calorie dinner should be both filling and light. Fresh vegetables (even steamed or lightly cooked), lean meats such as chicken or fish, beans, tofu, and a small portion of whole-grain bread are great for dinner. If you need something sweet for dessert, have a bowl of fresh fruit.

Now, for the things you *shouldn't* eat:

Diet Trap 1: High Calorie Additions

Most people start with the right idea for dinner, like fresh steamed vegetables, but then pile on unnecessary calories by adding creamy dressings, cheese, mayo, or margarine. For salads, use low-fat dressings, and if you're cooking vegetables, go easy on the grease. If you must fry, use olive oil—it's both light and healthy.

Diet Trap 2: Finishing Your Food

We all grew up with mom telling us to clean our plates, but we're all grown up now, so it's time to leave that idea behind. Listen to your body's cues, and if you don't want to eat any more, don't—put the leftovers in the garbage where they belong, instead of your stomach.

Diet Trap 3: No Starters

Appetizers aren't just mozzarella sticks and onion rings. One great way to improve the level of satisfaction and satiation you get from your low-calorie dinner is to incorporate healthy starters, such as soup or light salad.

Diet Trap 4: No Variety

Once you know the best and most easily prepared foods for dinner, such as chicken, it's important not to overdo them. If you have chicken every day, you'll get bored of it, setting yourself up for a binge. Make sure you incorporate variety in your diet plan; making a schedule for next week's dinners before you go grocery shopping is a good way to do this.

59

Banana Diet – One of the Simplest Ways to Lose Weight If You Do It Right

Bananas have always been popular, as a great, convenient healthy snack, but they've recently become a weight loss craze. The supposedly-miraculous Banana Diet first gained momentum in Japan, thanks to an endorsement by a local celebrity, and from there it's spread rapidly around the world. Overweight people are eating bananas by the dozen, hoping to shed those pounds as easily as bananas shed their peels. Here, we'll take a closer look at the banana diet, and examine whether it can really help you lose weight fast.

The Banana Diet Fad

One of the greatest appeals of the banana diet is its incredible convenience. After a mandatory breakfast of fresh bananas and water, you can eat whatever you want for the rest of the day, provided you a) eat a banana before every meal, b) eat dinner by 8 pm, c) have no dessert after dinner, and d) avoid ice cream, dairy products, and all beverages except water, including alcohol. According to dieticians Hitoshi and Sumiko Watanabe, that's all you need to do in order to lose weight rapidly. You can even have a sweet snack in the afternoon.

The Reality

It sounds great, but we need to burst the banana bubble—there are no weight loss miracles. Bananas have no secret weight loss properties. To lose weight, you can't escape the simple truth—you need to burn more calories than you consume.

The Benefits of Bananas

Like most other fruits, bananas are nutritious, and form a healthy component of a successful weight-loss diet. They're an excellent source of energy and, because of their high dietary fiber, they leave you feeling full. They're also a rich source of potassium and vitamin B6, two vital nutrients. But, sadly, a banana-rich diet has no extraordinary weight loss benefits.

Limitations of the Banana Diet

If you eat calorie-rich and unhealthy foods, you can have all the bananas you want, but you won't lose weight. Bananas don't offer you any protein, either, and without protein, even the rich fiber content of bananas won't leave you feeling completely full after breakfast. You'll be hungry again in no time, unless you supplement your breakfast with eggs, lean meat, light dairy, or beans.

The Diet Solution

Science has also demonstrated time and again that specialized, drastic diets don't work as effective long-term weight loss solutions. To rid yourself of excess weight consistently and maintain your healthy goal weight, you need to make sustainable lifestyle changes, including incorporating exercise into your routine.

The Verdict

By all means, have a banana or two, as long as you're not expecting any miracles! If you blend your bananas with low-fat yogurt and ice, you'll have a tasty breakfast smoothie, rich in lean protein and healthy carbohydrates. A banana is also an excellent workout snack, offering instant energy and replenishing the potassium you lost through sweat.

If you want to lose weight and achieve better health, try to consume a combination of fruit, instead of concentrating solely on bananas. Different colored fruits offer different health benefits, and all of them are effective components of a weight loss diet.

60

How to Lose Weight from Your Hips in Less Than a Month

If you want to lose weight from your hips, first you must understand that men's and women's bodies are programmed to store fat differently. For men, belly fat is a major concern; for women, it's the hips. If you want to lose weight from your hips, you should be prepared for a disciplined approach to diet and exercise. Yes, both are equally important; you can't get away with simply doing exercises to tone your hips, while eating whatever you want. By the same token, you can't follow a diet to take weight off your hips without doing any exercise—not if you want to see results, at any rate.

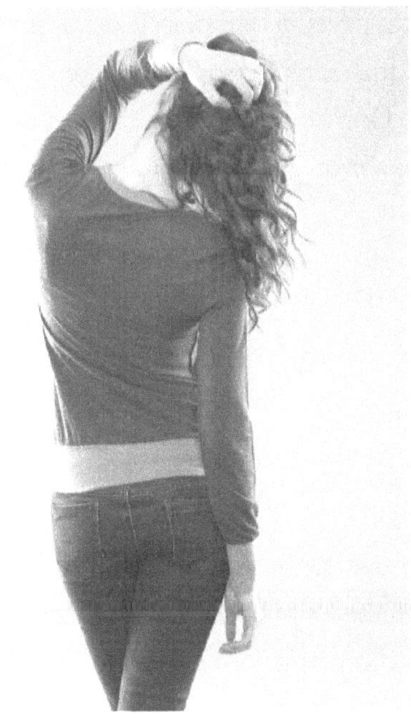

Why Diet and Exercise?

There's no natural method to target excess fat in one particular part of the body. If your objective is to reduce hip fat, you need to lose all your excess weight. Once that fat is gone, you can use exercise to target certain areas of your body, like your hips, to give them a tighter, leaner look.

A Weight Loss Diet Program

Start by replacing processed and instant foods with wholesome, freshly prepared meals. Sugar-rich sweets, oily snacks, burgers and sweetened drinks only pile on the calories, and they're absorbed so rapidly by your body that you quickly end up feeling hungry again, causing you to overeat. However, whole wheat and grains, fruits, and vegetables are complex carbohydrates, low in calories and high in fiber. They keep your body full for longer, and since they're more difficult to digest, they'll improve your body's metabolic rate.

Lean proteins such as chicken or fish, eggs, beans, lentils, nuts, and low-fat milk and dairy are also essential components of a weight loss diet. They, too, keep you feeling full, and help develop lean muscle mass. If you have wholesome meals, you won't overeat or indulge in fatty, sugary snacks, causing you to lose weight and reduce hip fat quickly. Don't forget to drink lots of water, and sleep—hydration and rest are essential to a properly functioning metabolism.

Hip Exercises

Toning your hips might not help you lose weight in that specific area, but it'll help avoid sagging skin and give you the lean, tight look you've always wanted. And the more toned your muscles are, the faster your metabolism is, and the more calories you'll burn every day.

Your hip region consists of three muscle groups: hip flexors, butt muscles, and groin muscles. Exercises like stair climbing, leg raises and lifts, and squats help tone these muscles. Incorporating some form of cardio into your workout is also a must; it'll help you burn even more calories and drop that hip fat quickly. With a consistent diet and exercise plan, you'll be able to lose weight off your hips in a matter of weeks!

61

Weight Loss and Fitness for Women in Their 30s – 4 Simple Facts Revealed

If you just hit your thirties, don't worry—you're still a young lady, and don't let anyone tell you otherwise! That's not just an inspirational mantra; science is on your side, too. Physiologically speaking, there's nothing you could achieve at 25 but can't at 32. You can still get fit, lose weight fast, and build your ideal body. However, you do need to acknowledge that your body is going through some changes, but as long as you're aware of them and act accordingly, you can still reach your goals. Weight loss and fitness has no age limit.

1. Understanding the Changes

To begin with, your natural metabolic rate is a bit slower than it was ten years ago, which means that, on average, your body burns fewer calories than it used to. A woman's body also begins to experience hormonal changes in her thirties. Skin elasticity begins to fall, and tiny wrinkles begin to appear on your face; skin renewal is also slower. These changes won't be drastic or sudden, but if you're in your thirties, this process has already begun, and you'll need to take some corrective measures to stay young-looking and healthy while you lose weight. Apart from a good skin care routine, it's crucial for you to maintain a healthy diet in the coming years.

2. Guess What? Exercise!

Exercise is essential for anyone who wants to lose weight and keep it off; it's no less important for you as you make your way through your thirties. Apart from helping you get slim, exercise—especially some form of strength training—will improve your muscle tone, boost the elasticity of your skin, and improve blood circulation. If you're facing a lot of stress at work, the endorphins released through regular exercise will help counter its effects. Women who are planning a pregnancy in their thirties especially need regular exercise, as it affects the health of their fetus.

3. Diet

As mentioned previously, the other part of your fitness and weight loss plan is diet. Try to eliminate junk food as much as you can, and other unhealthy habits like drinking and smoking. Other than weight gain, there are countless other negative health impacts associated with these habits, especially over thirty. Drinking enough water will help flush these toxins from your body and keep your skin healthy and hydrated.

Divide up your meals and snacks so you eat small meals 5–6 times a day. This keeps your metabolism running at peak performance. A diet rich in fruits and vegetables helps cut calories and supplies you with vital minerals, vitamins, and antioxidants. Lean protein keeps your muscles strong, and remember to get enough calcium; milk and milk products have them in abundance. Women in their thirties with calcium deficiencies may soon begin to experience arthritic symptoms.

4. Controlling Your Enthusiasm

Motivation is excellent, but rein in your enthusiasm and don't go overboard with these changes, if you want sustainable health and weight loss success. If you change too many things too quickly, it'll be difficult to maintain them, and you're likely to slip back into old habits. Work on one thing at a time, and try to make it a part of your life, not just your weight loss plan.

62

5 Crucial Diet Tips for Business Travelers – How to Travel and Remain Slim

If you travel frequently for business, the combination of work stress, disrupted routine, business dinners and food temptations put you at high risk to gain weight. If you're seeing these changes in yourself, weight loss is likely on your mind. However, if you're prepared to follow these tips, there's hope for change, even as you travel.

1. It Is No Drought!

Water is one of the easiest things to forget among the stresses, pressures and distractions of traveling. But when water isn't an essential part of your travel diet plan, your dehydrated body may interpret thirst as hunger, causing you to overeat—not to mention that dehydration slows your metabolism significantly. So carry a bottle with you when you leave your hotel in the morning, and set reminders throughout the day to drink.

2. Healthy Snacks Exist Even Far Away

When you're traveling, with only a small window of time to grab lunch, you'll probably stop at the first drive-thru you see and wolf down a burger, fries, and soda. But in that same limited time frame, you could stop at a grocery store instead, and pick up some fruit, nuts, and a low-calorie tuna salad. Even if they don't amount to a full lunch, they should be enough to drive the hunger pangs away and help you resist the temptation of the drive-thru. If you know you're going to be very pressed for time during your next business trip, pack plenty of non-perishable, healthy snacks from home.

3. Be Your Own Chef

If you're going to be on the road for a while, you'll probably be checked in at an extended-stay hotel, the kind that gives you a small kitchenette or microwave. This is ideal for the dieting traveler. Stock up on healthy cereal like oatmeal. You can even buy healthy frozen meals which simply need to be heated up. Your hotel's in-house chef will probably be more than happy to accommodate your weight loss plan, if they don't already have a menu for health-conscious travelers.

4. Will You Lose Weight With Booze?

Drinking is another obstacle for the dieting traveler. You must control your alcohol intake, if you're serious about your goals. Not only does alcohol have a lot of calories (and cocktails are even worse) it leads to overeating through loss of inhibitions. So sip your drink slowly, and limit yourself to one or two drinks. If you want a cocktail, Bloody Marys and Tom Collins are the lightest in terms of calories, between 130–150 calories each.

5. The Devastating Daily Binge

Of course, you don't want to miss the cultural experience of eating out, even if you're trying to follow a healthy diet plan. Make sure you're only bingeing occasionally, though, and that the majority of your meals are healthy. Many restaurants, even those overseas, have great-tasting low-calorie meals, so take advantage.

63

Diets and Weight Loss Secrets – 3 Reasons Why Your Weight Loss Diet is Not Working

If you're serious about losing weight, but have been dieting for ages without seeing any results, you're probably getting pretty frustrated. Time to sit back and examine the reasons behind your failure; chances are some of these bad habits have snuck in and disrupted your weight loss efforts.

1. Diet Traps

Considering the number of weight loss myths and misleadingly marketed diet products, we won't be surprised if you've fallen for one of these. Some of the most common pitfalls are manufactured fat-free foods. You see this proclamation on the packages of cookies, dressings and jams, and even ice cream. But losing weight doesn't involve cutting fat from your diet; you need to cut *calories*. To compensate for the lack of taste when fat is omitted, however, the manufacturers of these products load them with flavored syrups, sugar, salt or starch. Empty calories, in other words, which are counterproductive to weight loss.

There are other weight loss food categories people tend to fall for, such as fat-free yogurt and fruit juices. Both have high sugar contents, packing you full of calories without satisfying. While 100% fruit juices are healthier, they still don't contain the fiber of whole fruit, and can't fill you up. If you want to make low-fat yogurt a part of your diet, choose a variety which is also low in added sugar and calories.

2. Eating For Reasons Other Than Hunger

We all do this every now and then, but some people fall into this pattern more than others. No one reaches for a salad when they're stressed! If you get caught in the 'comfort food' trap every time you're feeling stressed, lonely, or emotional, you'll only end up feeling guilty, which makes everything worse. Rather than rushing to your favorite hamburger place or ice cream parlor the next time you're feeling down, try exercise instead. It's a far more productive way of relieving stress. You don't have to pump iron in a gym for an hour. Just go out for a quiet walk to a nice place, do some yoga, or even meditate.

3. A Large Dinner

After staying committed to a strict diet all day, avoiding junk snacks and meals, you might end up skipping a meal or two, thinking you can make it up with a big dinner. But nighttime, when your body begins to slow down and prepare for sleep, is the worst time to pack in the calories, and can completely destroy all that hard work with excess food. And a full stomach can negatively affect your sleep, further slowing your metabolism. Move your focus to having four to five small meals during the day, with a light dinner a few hours before bed.

64

Weight Loss for a Size Zero Figure – 3 Must Know Facts

Weight loss is no longer a concern restricted to overweight women. Even those who have a Body Mass Index (BMI) in the normal range are still striving to lose pounds. It's not hard to understand why; simply turn on the television or open a magazine. The modern concept of beauty is a stick-thin, 'size zero' figure. As a woman, you've surely heard that beauty is not skin deep, and neither is it restricted to your dress size. You might have even said it yourself. Words are all well and good, but deep down, can you deny you still feel that a size zero figure would give you that extra edge of pride and confidence? If so, read on.

1. Size Zero Or Good Health?

Experts know this fascination with 'size zero,' and the extreme measures women resort are willing to implement to achieve it, can lead to tragic consequences. The choice for most women, though, is "size zero or good health"; even "size zero or long life." When you go on an extreme diet to achieve and maintain an unnaturally skinny figure, you run the risk of developing serious osteoporosis early in life. Women are susceptible to bone density problems to begin with, but the risk increases exponentially for women with no body fat and underdeveloped muscles. According to researchers, some fat mass is crucial for bone density.

Obsession with a skinny body can also lead to anorexia, body dysmorphic disorders, and bulimia, all of which can be fatal. In the past few years, three top models—two Uruguayan sisters and a Brazilian woman—have died of malnutrition due to anorexia. They were all under twenty-five years of age, reportedly surviving on a few pieces of fruit and vegetables a day.

2. Appreciate Your Body Type

Most women simply don't have the body type to achieve a size zero. Some have a wider bone structure and are naturally more solidly built. If that's the case, you have a better chance at good health and glowing, vibrant skin than petite women who've starved the life out of them for extreme weight loss. So, play to your best features, and learn to love yourself!

3. The Right Kind of Role Models

The next time you see a socialite or actress like Nicole Richie or Kareena Kapoor flaunting their size zero figures and winning stares of admiration, try to tear your eyes away and look for other role models. Former Miss World Gul Panag hasn't minced words on the matter: "Looking thin is like being a poster girl for sickness and bad health. I believe it's more important to be fit than be thin and look sick." There are plenty of other beauty queens and actresses who openly endorse this view, and, thankfully, it's catching on. Many modeling agencies and famous fashion brands have gone as far as openly rejecting overly skinny poster girl applicants.

It's no longer necessary to be a size zero to be Miss Universe, feature on the cover of Vogue, be admired on the red carpet, or simply be considered beautiful. The trends are changing; it's much more glamorous to be proud of your body, maintain a healthy weight for *you*, and seek better levels of fitness and health.

65

How to Lose Fat from Upper Arms and Achieve a Lean Figure

Heavy upper arms are a common problem among women, and not just women who are overweight. Even women who are slim and have a healthy BMI face this problem, and are desperate to find a way to lose fat from their upper arms.

If you're in the same boat, you need to know that, although the body stores fat unevenly in specific areas of the body, there's no non-surgical method to melt fat from those targeted areas. You have to lose weight by burning more calories than you consume and lose fat from everywhere on your body, including your problem areas.

Importance of Muscle Toning

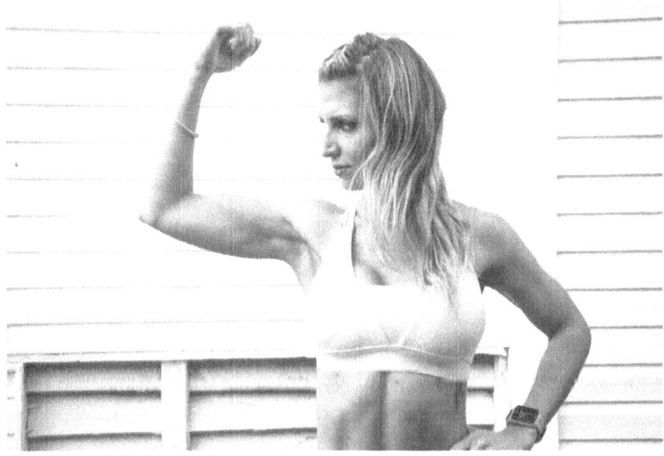

But there are ways to tone your muscles in specific areas of your body, such as your arms. When you tone your arms and develop lean muscle, they'll start to look tighter, achieving the lean look you want. Developing more lean muscle improves your metabolism, too, helping you lose weight fast and acquire a slim, hourglass figure. To start you off, here are two useful exercises to tone your arms. All you'll need is a set of light dumbbells (or full soup cans or water bottles, if you don't want to go out and buy a set of weights). Try to repeat this routine 2–3 times a week to tone your arms.

Overhead Press

This exercise works your triceps, biceps, and shoulders. Stand straight with your feet shoulder-width apart and contract your abs. Weights in hand, hold your arms up and out from your sides at shoulder level. Bend your elbows at a 90 degree angle, with your palms facing forward. This is your starting position.

Now, lift the dumbbells or weight straight overhead until your arms are fully extended beside your ears. Pause, then rotate your wrists so your palms and forearms face behind you. Hold for a few seconds, then lower your weights straight down to chin level, keeping your elbows as close to your body as possible, and hold for a few seconds again. Raise your arms back up, and rotate so your palms are once again facing forward, then return to starting position. Try two sets of 15–25 repetitions each.

Cross Punches

This exercise also works your abs, as well as your arms and shoulders. Stand once again with your feet shoulder-width apart. Tuck your arms in, elbows bent and palms brushing your sides. Now, pivot on your right hip, rotating your right hip and shoulder toward your left, extending your arm out for a punch. You don't have to punch hard, so don't swing your body with a jerk or thrust your arm out; move with control. Repeat the movement with the other arm in the opposite direction. This completes one rep. Perform two sets of this exercise, 15–25 repetitions each.

If you're concerned that strength training will give you a bulky, muscular look, remember that, without artificial hormones, that's physically impossible. Toning your arms will give you lean muscle mass, which is crucial to lose fat from your upper arms and all over your body, giving you the slim, shapely look you want.

66

Is Your 2018 Weight Loss Plan a Sustainable One – Check It Out!

Many people began this year with the goal of losing weight. A lot of them are even aware that, mathematically, weight loss is a simple game of calories in/calories out. If you burn 2,000 calories a day, and consume 1,800, your body will make up for that deficit by burning 200 calories worth of fat. No expert will argue with that. The challenge is finding a sustainable weight loss plan to keep you in a consistent calorie deficit, and improve your health at the same time.

Think Long-Term

A drastic, calorie-chopping diet isn't the answer. Extreme weight loss will damage your health and energy levels, and it's temporary, lasting only as long as your drastic diet. You need a sustainable plan that ideally combines both diet and exercise. Only with a consistent, long-term plan will you be able to achieve and maintain a healthy body.

Be Practical

A sustainable plan means setting practical diet targets. If you love sweets, and your diet plan requires you to give them up cold-turkey, you're setting yourself up for suffering and failure. Instead, cut down on sweets gradually, and have a strategy to deal with cravings when they strike, such as having healthy alternatives like fruit on hand. If you can substitute instant, processed foods with more wholesome, fiber-rich and natural foods, to whatever extent, you're on the right track.

Incorporate Any Exercise

As any expert will tell you, exercise is also very important for fast weight loss. Once again, you need to remain practical. Keep your interests and current levels of fitness in mind, and set your exercise targets accordingly. For instance, if you're out of shape, but love to dance, why not sign up for a beginner-level Zumba class, instead of slogging it out in the gym? You can also play a sport, go bicycling, swimming, running, or even go out for a brisk walk. Any form of aerobic exercise will tone your muscles and burn calories. As your body adapts to the routine over a few months, you can raise the level of challenge. Most experts agree two-and-a-half hours of exercise a week—or half an hour of exercise, five days a week—will keep you fit and strong.

Be sure, however, to consult a physician before incorporating any exercise in your weight loss plan, especially if you've been sedentary for several years. If you have any history of medical problems or injuries, your doctor can make recommendations to keep you healthy and safe on your journey.

The Right Mental Attitude

Mind over matter, right? A good mental attitude is also very important. Stay patient, and don't get obsessed with the scale; give yourself two months to see substantial change. And if you find your weight loss plan isn't working for you, simply alter it according to your limitations and lifestyle, instead of giving up. The objective is long-term change, so gradual progress is fine. Whatever weight loss plan you follow, make sure you reward yourself for meeting your goals, with treats such as a shopping trip or massage.

67

How to Lose 10 Pounds Fast with 10 Minutes of Exercise

So, you want to lose ten pounds fast this season, but you don't have much time to spare for consistent exercise. Plenty of other people are in the same boat, but the good news is you can still achieve your weight loss goals in only two ten minute exercise sessions a day. If global political leaders, film stars, and CEOs can do it, so can you!

The Magic of Short Spells of Exercise

If you want to lose ten pounds, can commit to regulating your diet, and are consistent with a total of twenty minutes of exercise per day, there's no reason why you can't lose ten pounds in as little as two to three months! Most people think exercise has to be done in one continuous session, for an hour or more, to provide any real benefit. That's simply not true! Whether you complete your exercise in one session, two sessions, or three, you'll still burn the same number of calories. Put it this way—if you want to do sixty jumping jacks, it doesn't matter if you do them in one single session, or do twenty at breakfast, lunch, and dinner. Either way, at the end of the day, you've still done sixty jumping jacks.

The easiest way for you to begin is to pick two exercises you have the space, capability, and equipment for, and do a ten-minute session of each per day. Here are some ideas:

Jumping Rope

With just a jump rope and a little bit of empty space, even a moderate session of jumping rope can burn 100–110 calories in ten minutes. You'll be hard pressed to find a more efficient weight loss exercise. The best part? You don't even need the rope! It's slightly less effective, since you're not working with the weight and resistance of the rope, but you can jump in place and swing your arms as though you were working an invisible jump rope, which is great if you're really tight on space.

Climbing Stairs

Ten minutes on the stairs will help you burn 70–80 calories, and you don't even have to sprint up. Stair climbing engages your leg muscles and helps tone them. Toned muscles mean a better metabolism, which, as we all know, translates to further weight loss!

Stationary Bike and Treadmill

If you've got a stationary bike, set it right in front of your television. If you can ignore your couch and pedal away for ten minutes while your favorite show plays, you've just burned 60–70 calories. Hit the treadmill for the same amount of time, and you might even reach the 100-calorie mark.

Walking and Active Lifestyle

Brisk walking will help burn around 50 calories in ten minutes; dancing for as much time could burn over 70. But if nothing else is working, simply incorporating as much exercise as possible into your daily routine, by taking the stairs and parking at the opposite end of the lot, will help you burn 50–60 extra calories. And if you're a parent, get outside and play with your kids! You'll have fun and lose weight, too.

By combining twenty minutes of exercise with a healthy diet, you'll be able to lose ten pounds before summer is through!

68

Walk Off Your Pounds and Lose Weight Fast!

People are constantly on the lookout for a magic diet pill or groundbreaking weight loss secret, but in the process, they tend to forget that the best weight loss plans simply involve an increased emphasis on physical activities and healthier eating habits. And one of the most effective activities is one of the simplest: walking.

Set the Right Pace

You don't need to set off like a torpedo and tire yourself out in ten minutes, but a leisurely, meandering pace isn't going to help either. Walk at a moderately brisk pace you think you can maintain for half an hour; a speed of about 3–4 miles per hour is pretty good, but, especially if you've been sedentary for a long time, judge your pace by effort expended, not speed. You should be breathing slightly harder than normal and feel your body warming up, without panting or feeling fatigued.

Most medical experts recommend about thirty minutes per day, five days a week, of cardiovascular exercise to maintain good health. Walking might not seem terribly athletic, but it counts, and it burns about 100–165 calories per mile, depending on your weight. In thirty minutes of brisk walking, you could burn 200–300 calories.

How Much?

If you maintain this schedule five days a week, without altering your diet in any way, by the end of the month you'll lose 1–2 pounds. That means in six months, you'll have lost thirteen pounds! That's an excellent rate of weight loss, and shows just how effective walking is.

Walking vs Jogging

The myth persists among many people, though, that unless they go out jogging and end up sweaty and out of breath at the end, they won't burn enough calories to lose weight fast. In fact, there's a negligible difference in the number of calories brisk walking burns vs jogging per mile. What really matters is the amount of distance you cover. You can run hard for eight minutes and tire yourself out, but you still won't burn as many calories as someone who walked briskly for twenty minutes and covered more distance. Walking also puts you at less risk for impact-related injuries. For a person of average fitness, if your objective is simply to lose weight, walking is the more efficient workout.

Bringing Walking Into Your Life

The best news might be that the thirty minutes of walking per day you need for quick weight loss doesn't have to be done at one time. The cumulative exercise time is what really matters. So, if you're busy, just incorporate walking into your routine, by parking your car a block away, or walking to the grocery store. And of course, walking also tones your muscles, speeding your metabolism to burn more calories while you rest. It improves cardiovascular health, too, and your overall fitness, bone density, and cognitive health! Talk about a magic strategy to lose weight fast!

69

How to Lose 9 Pounds Fast – The Healthiest Recipe

Why nine pounds? Why not ten, or fifteen, or twenty? Nine is the highest of the single-digit numbers, and psychologically easy to achieve, but closest to ten, the lowest of the two-digit numbers, and so is a good initial target which will be easy to achieve.

If you're ready to lose nine pounds fast, you need to educate yourself to recognize and avoid the health food trap. There are *lots* of food items on the shelves of your neighborhood supermarket trying to pass themselves off as healthy, to trick you into buying them. Be smart, and take control of your choices! Even if it's a seemingly healthy salad dressing, processed food is not the answer.

The Problem Ingredients – Enemies of Losing Weight Fast

Most commercially manufactured dressings contain large quantities of HFCS (High Fructose Corn Syrup), which means that "healthy" dressing is actually loaded with sugar. Read the labels carefully, and you'll see how many dressings contain HFCS.

Not only that, most dressings also contain either refined canola oil or refined soybean oil. Some even contain both! But soybean oil contains way too many omega-6 fatty acids, and the oxidized polyunsaturated fats in both pose some serious health problems. None of these ingredients will help you achieve your weight loss goals.

There's a simple answer, though, if you still want to enjoy a tasteful, healthy salad to help you on your way to losing nine pounds fast: make your own dressing. You probably already have all the readily-available ingredients at home, and it takes less than ten minutes to make.

A Homemade Salad Dressing Recipe

Take a salad dressing container, and fill it with these ingredients:

- 1/3rd apple cider vinegar

- 1/3rd balsamic vinegar

- 1/3rd equal proportions of olive oil (extra virgin) and an oil blend enriched with Essential Fatty Acids (EFA), such as 'Udo's Choice'.

- Pinch of black pepper, garlic powder and onion powder

- 1–2 teaspoons of genuine 100% maple syrup

Shake to mix well, and you have your own healthy salad dressing. Your homemade version has none of the harmful ingredients of a commercial dressing, but lacks for nothing in terms of taste. In fact, you'll probably find that it tastes *better* than most other dressings you can buy at the store. The best part is you can adapt this recipe to your individual taste, by altering the proportions of herbs and maple syrup.

The Health Advantages

This recipe has a significant quantity of unrefined polyunsaturated oils, as well as the perfect balance of omega-3 and omega-6 fatty acids. The EFA blend is what provides this; just make sure the one you buy is cold-processed, as heating essential fatty acids not only destroys some of their nutritional value, but can also cause the formation of dangerous free radicals.

So, now you know how a seemingly insignificant salad dressing could influence your weight loss efforts. You don't have to be a victim of marketing schemes; a little bit of education and effort is all you need to make responsible choices, and achieve your goals, better fitness, and longer life in the process!

70

Finding Ways to Lose Weight Fast – Can Pilates Help Me Lose Weight Fast?

Along with yoga, Pilates has become a very popular form of exercise. People come to a Pilates class with a variety of expectations, most of which involve losing weight. So, how does Pilates compare to other forms of exercise?

Is Pilates The Best Way For Weight Loss?

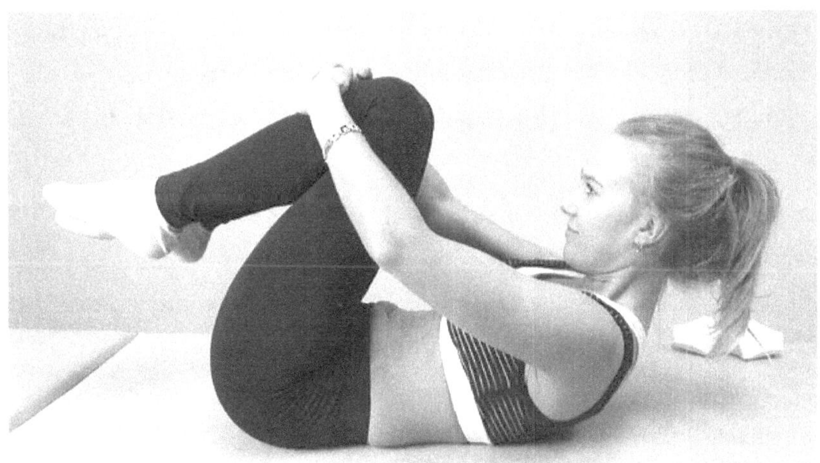

There are many health and fitness objectives for which Pilates is one of the most effective exercise systems available; unfortunately, losing weight fast isn't one of them. While Pilates still helps you burn a significant number of calories, it simply can't compare to traditional cardiovascular workouts such as jogging, cycling, and jumping rope. And since losing weight is a simple equation of burning more calories than you consume, Pilates isn't the most efficient way to lose weight fast. It does, however, aid fitness and weight loss in several ways.

Calories Comparison

For a 145-pound person, an hour of brisk cycling or jogging can burn 500–550 calories. A run cranks that number up to over 850 calories, and an hour of jumping rope burns 600–650 calories. But an hour of beginner's Pilates only burns around 250 calories, an intermediate class accounts for nearly 340 calories, and an advanced level around 420 calories. So, for pure calories burned, Pilates just doesn't stack up.

The Indirect Weight Loss Advantages

In spite of the above, Pilates can be a very useful part of any exercise regimen, as it has some crucial indirect weight loss advantages. Pilates improves your posture, flexibility, muscle tone and lean muscle mass, and core strength. It also improves your overall energy level, physical fitness, and sense of well-being. These advantages can lead to a dramatic improvement in the rest of your exercise regimen, whether it's running, cycling, or brisk walking. You'll have more stamina, burn more calories, and be less susceptible to injury.

More lean muscle mass means a better metabolic rate, even while at rest. Pilates helps change your body shape significantly, even if your weight doesn't change much. When you have more lean muscle, your posture improves, making you look taller and slimmer and giving you confidence. After doing Pilates regularly, people have reported a lot of positive feedback from their colleagues, friends, and family. On the subject of lean muscle—Pilates can be a good muscle-toning substitute for those who simply can't stomach weight training.

Like any other exercise regimen, Pilates isn't a magic cure. You'll have to practice consistently for a few weeks before you begin to see results. Make sure you regulate your diet and eat healthier while you do Pilates, too, if you're serious about weight loss.

71

I Want to Lose Weight Fast! is It Possible with a Busy Lifestyle?

Busy people who sit at a desk for most of the day are at high risk to become overweight or obese. The body gets softer, the clothes get tighter, and one day, the realization dawns. You want to burn all that ugly fat away. You know you need exercise to lose weight fast, but how can you find the time?

Think About Your Diet

What do you eat on an average day, and why? Have you been skipping meals, eating irregularly, and ignoring the health content of your meals due to pressure at work? Do you binge when emotional? Is your diet full of sodas, snacks, and processed foods, because you're short on time? Once you've determined the problems with your diet, and what's causing them, you can start working on the solutions, and build a better diet.

The Right Kind of Changes

Now you know the problem with your diet, but the circumstances causing it aren't going to change, and sudden, extreme dietary changes simply aren't possible. That's all right; those sorts of changes aren't even recommended for weight loss. People who go on drastic diets aren't able to sustain them, putting them into a vicious cycle of weight loss and weight gain, which is neither healthy nor advisable. Small, sustainable changes can still help you start losing weight quickly, but will also keep it off for good.

Healthy Snacks

First, start snacking healthy. Throw out those bags of chips and chocolate, and substitute fresh fruit or whole grain cereal and milk. With just a few portions of fresh fruit and vegetables a day, you can keep those calorie-laden snacks from becoming a temptation. Your energy levels will improve, and you'll feel fuller for longer. And picking up healthy snacks instead of junk won't cost you any extra time.

Drink More Water

Eight to ten glasses of water per day prevents dehydration, which slows your metabolism. Dehydration also tricks your body into thinking it's hungry, when it's really just thirsty, leading to unnecessary consumption of calories.

Passive Exercise

The phrase may sound like an oxymoron, but passive exercise incorporates calorie-burning activities which easily fit into your daily routine, without requiring any special effort. Take the stairs instead of the elevator, park your car two blocks away from the office, or a brief jog to the supermarket instead of a stroll are all examples of passive exercise. These small efforts can yield big results in extra calories burned.

We know you want to lose weight fast, but don't go *too* fast. Your weight loss effort will be far more productive in the long run if it's consistent, and achieved with healthy, sustainable lifestyle changes.

72

Want to Lose Weight Fast? is Your Grocery Shopping Sabotaging Your Weight Loss Plans?

It might seem strange to think that a mundane task like grocery shopping could be sabotaging your weight loss plan, but if you think about it, the things you buy at the grocery store form the foundation of your daily diet. This has nothing to do with the brands or products you buy, and everything to do with the way you shop.

The first mistake most people make is ignoring their list completely. Why even make a grocery list, if you're going to throw it out the window at the first sight of a bargain? But your grocery list details all the things that are essential to feed you and your family and run your household. If that buy-two-get-three "healthy, fat-free yogurt" deal isn't on your list to begin with, you probably don't need it. And that reduced-price cereal could very well be reduced quality, too.

At the opposite end of the scale, if you're sticking too closely to your shopping list, you could be missing out on other, better options. It's understandable; when you get comfortable eating the same food month after month, you put it down on your list without thinking. Take a look around, and you might spot a fortified whole-wheat pasta two shelves above your usual, low-fiber brand. Be a bit adventurous, and you might just better your quality of life.

The final, and by far the most common, mistake is overstocking your pantry. It's good to have a little extra, in case the unexpected strikes, but you're not shopping to survive a nuclear war or a biblical flood. More often than not, the items you tend to stock in bulk are those reduced-price, too-good-to-pass up bargains. Better to pass, instead of overstocking things you don't want. If it's in your house, you're probably going to end up eating it, and that's not really part of your plan, is it?

What can you do to avoid these shopping mistakes? First, educate yourself, and become a smarter consumer. Be vigilant when it comes to labels—the nutritional content, the ingredients, and the expiration date. Don't be seduced by unbelievable prices or fancy packaging.

The second piece of advice might sound a bit strange, but it works—shop on a full stomach. You'll be much less tempted by all those unnecessary but delicious-sounding discounted food items, and you can keep your weight loss plan on track. Happy shopping!

73

Can You Lose Weight and Get a Flat Tummy with Laxative Tea – Read These 4 Facts!

Weight loss is hard work; if you've been searching for an elusive secret to losing weight quickly and easily, you're not alone. Sadly, there is no such secret; only a lot of gimmicks aimed at taking advantage of desperate people, and many of them are even dangerous. Laxative teas are one of these, so before you set out to buy one, read on.

The Weight Loss Caused by Laxative Teas

Many people *have* lost weight with herbal laxative teas, but that weight loss isn't healthy or consistent, and isn't even from excess body fat. Rather, what people lose is vital water. The water is lost through diarrhea, which is what laxative tea causes, the intensity of which varies with the amount you consume and your body's tolerance. Apart from diarrhea, herbal laxative tea can also cause digestion problems, abdominal cramps, vomiting, weakness, and, in some extreme cases, death.

The Dangers

Laxative teas don't cause real weight loss because they act in the large intestine, whereas most of your body's excess calories and fat are stored in the small intestine. The effects of these teas on the large intestine are quite destructive, which is why they cause the painful and dangerous symptoms listed above. If you continue to consume these laxative teas over a long period of time, your colon will become sluggish, and might even lose the ability to produce normal bowel movements. As a result, you'll need more and more tea to keep yourself from becoming constipated, and could become dependent on them, leading to fatal consequences. The chronic diarrhea caused by laxative tea can also lead to malabsorption and loss of vital nutrients, such as potassium.

Constipation Relief and Detoxification

Many people use herbal laxative teas not only to lose weight, but for constipation relief and supposed detoxification benefits. There are better, safer alternatives for both of these benefits out there, though—and besides, there's no conclusive study proving these teas are any good for detoxification.

The Misleading 'Herbal' Label

Often, people are taken in by the "herbal," label, thinking it means "natural and healthy." But nature is full of powerful herbs which can be very dangerous, if consumed in large enough quantities. The typical ingredients of laxative teas are senna leaf, rhubarb root, cascara, aloe, buckthorn and castor oil. All these herbs are powerful, and can have serious side effects when taken in the quantities laxative teas contain. Rhubarb root and senna leaf are recognized by the FDA as especially dangerous.

Ultimately, the only real weight loss solution is the combination of a healthy and balanced diet and sufficient exercise. If these aren't working for you, see your physician—you may have a medical condition causing your excess weight gain.

74

You Can Lose Weight Fast and Easy with a Balanced Diet – Follow These 3 Amazingly Simple Tips

A balanced diet is crucial for healthy and consistent weight loss, and eventual weight maintenance. Most people have heard this *ad nauseum*, but not everyone understands what a balanced diet means, and how it's achieved. The problem is that, with all the drastic, restrictive, and ultimately ineffective fad diets around, proper dietary information often gets lost in all the noise.

The Meaning of a Balanced Diet

A healthy and balanced diet is a nutrient-rich diet, or, in other words, a diet consisting of food items offering high numbers of nutrients and fewer calories. It's also a varied diet, since every food has its own nutritional limitations, and ignoring any particular food group can cause serious nutritional deficiencies. When a diet is nutrient-rich and varied, it's balanced. This sort of diet will keep you feeling healthy, keep your metabolism high, and lead to sustainable weight loss. But, if a healthy diet is so simple and straightforward, why have fad diets become so popular?

Why Fad Diets?

Mainly because they offer a few irresistible attractions. First, they're short-term diets, so the sacrifices and inconveniences don't last more than a few weeks at best. Second, fad diets promise fast weight loss in the extreme. What you might lose in ten months with exercise and a balanced diet, a fad diet promises you'll lose in six weeks. And many people fall for the gimmick, risking dehydration and severe health problems in the process. If you're lucky enough to escape these side effects, there's one problem with fad diets that's inescapable—the weight you lose always comes back.

The Essential Foods

Fruits and vegetables – High in vital nutrients and fiber, and low in calories, fruits and vegetables have the power to satisfy your hunger without loading your body with excess calories. A healthy diet should consist of a bowl of fruit every day, and a full serving of vegetables at every meal.

Lean meats, eggs, beans, and lentils – These vital sources of protein are crucial to build muscles, and, like fruits and vegetables, keep you fuller longer, preventing you from overeating.

Milk and other dairy products – Milk and milk-based products like cheese and yogurt contain a substantial amount of vital protein, and are also an important source of calcium and vitamins. To keep calories in check, choose low-fat milk and milk products. Try to consume a glass of milk, a serving of yogurt, and a small portion of cheese every day.

Cereals, potatoes, and bread – These foods are essential sources of carbohydrates, your body's main fuel. They should account for a third of your everyday calorie consumption. Stick to unrefined varieties, like whole wheat bread and pasta, and whole grains. They're high in fiber and digest more slowly, keeping you full and speeding up your metabolism through the digestion process.

75

How to Slim Down Your Hips and Thighs

Many people first realize they need to lose weight when they look in the mirror, and see that specific parts of their body are sticking out rather unappealingly. Hardly anyone gains weight uniformly; your excess weight may be concentrated around your stomach, hips, thighs, underarms, and even your face. But no matter how out of shape you might be, it's possible to achieve lean and strong thighs and great hips.

All-round Weight Loss the Only Way

If you want to lose weight quickly from your hips and thighs, and reshape them, you need to know there's no exercise method in the world to help you lose weight from specific areas of the body. Weight loss is an overall process, accomplished by consuming fewer calories than you burn in a day. In order to do this, you need to regulate your diet and incorporate cardiovascular exercise into your routine. When you lose weight, you'll lose it from everywhere, though not uniformly. Fat will disappear from some areas of the body quickly, and be more stubborn in others. There's no way to control this process more specifically.

Shaping Your Hips and Thighs

However, by losing weight fast, you won't necessarily obtain a good shape by default. To get those perfectly shaped hips and thighs, you need to tone those muscles with specific strength-building exercises. Once your muscles develop, they'll give your hips and thighs a lean, long and shapely form. If you're a woman, don't worry—you won't end up looking overly muscular, as your body doesn't produce enough testosterone to develop bulky muscles.

The Right Exercises

There are several different exercises you can do to tone the hips and thighs. Two very effective exercise systems known for producing excellent results in these areas are Power Yoga and Pilates. Both have specific, effective exercises to tone your hips and thighs, but since they are total body workouts, they'll tone other parts of your body, too, improving your overall physical health, balance, posture, and core strength. Leg lifts, squats, and crunches are also very effective at toning your hips and thighs.

The Right Guidance

Whatever exercise system you choose, it's important to get proper guidance. There's a correct form and method for every exercise, and your levels of difficulty need to be build up gradually as your fitness improves, in carefully planned steps. To do Pilates and/or Power Yoga successfully, you need to already be at a reasonable fitness level.

In conclusion, the only way to lose that excess weight around your hips and thighs is with a healthy diet, cardiovascular exercise, and targeted muscle strengthening. These three strategies will come together to give you the shape you've always wanted.

76

How to Get Perfect V-Cut Abs

There's a lot of conflicting information out there on getting sculpted, defined abs. Many 'experts' talk about the subject as though they're sharing some closely-guarded secret. But six-pack abs aren't the result of a secret formula; by following some simple steps, you should be able to lose weight fast and achieve that sculpted v-cut you've always wanted.

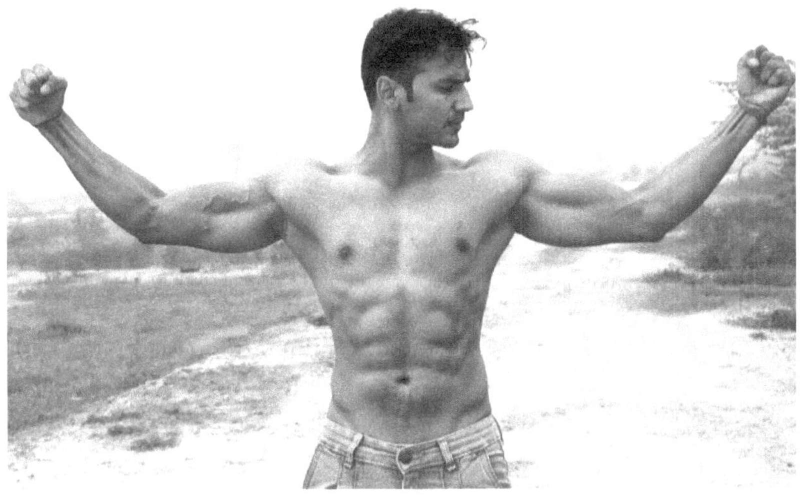

The Right Diet

The most important factor in getting that six-pack is an excellent diet. Your body fat needs to be at a minimum, otherwise it won't matter how strong your abs are—they won't show under that layer of fat. Burning fat is the same as losing weight; it requires that you consume fewer calories than you burn over the course of the day.

Fruits and Vegetables

To lower your calorie consumption, start by cutting junk food, sugary sweets, and alcohol. Whenever you feel like snacking, pick up a healthy choice like fruit or almonds. Fruits and vegetables will be one of the most important food groups for you, filling you up with healthy fiber and vital nutrients without excess calories. And once you get used to eating fruits and vegetables instead of chips and chocolate, you'll find you're addicted!

Lean Proteins

Your diet also needs to be rich in lean protein, through grains, lentils, beans, milk products, eggs, and lean meats such as chicken or fish. Your body needs this protein to repair and build your muscles after exercise. A protein-rich meal keeps you fuller and prevents you from overeating. If you don't get enough protein, you won't be able to develop your muscles or improve your metabolism. In other words, you can forget about that six-pack.

Cardiovascular Exercises

A good diet is better than half the battle, but an effective exercise routine is just as important. Reducing your body fat percentage means actively burning those excess calories through cardiovascular exercise. Try jogging, jumping rope, cycling or swimming three to five times a week, for at least half an hour at a time. No matter how much muscle-building you do, nothing burns calories as effectively as aerobic exercise.

Muscle Strengthening

Your exercise plan must also incorporate muscle toning and strengthening exercises, if you're serious about that six-pack. The higher your ratio of muscle mass, the faster your metabolism will be, and the more calories you'll burn. Besides, it's the muscle toning that will really sculpt that drool-worthy shape and make those abs stand out. Don't just focus on your abdominals, though; an effective muscle-strengthening exercise routine will tone your whole body. So, after your crunches, leg lifts, and other abdominal exercises, work in some squats, lunges, and pushups, too. All three develop your core strength, vital for strong abs and a fit body.

If you stick with these tips for eight to twelve weeks, there's nothing to prevent you from losing weight rapidly, and getting those six-pack abs you've always dreamed of.

77

Will Yoga Help You Lose Weight Fast?

Yoga offers several health benefits, such as improved flexibility, better strength, muscle toning and stress reduction. It makes you feel better about your body in general, and also reportedly improves your sense of mental well-being. But what many people want to know about is its effectiveness as a weight loss workout. If you want to lose weight fast, you want to know how the hard numbers add up.

The Ineffectiveness of Regular Yoga

Unfortunately, most forms of yoga, as the sole source of exercise, won't achieve significant weight loss. It doesn't raise your heart rate sufficiently and for long enough periods of time to work as a weight loss tool. On average, a one hour session of yoga burns about 160 calories for a 150 pound person, compared to 300 calories for a three mile-per-hour walk for the same period of time. The figures simply don't add up to significant calorie burn, particularly if you're a beginner who's new to fitness and has limited flexibility. However, if you're already reasonably fit, and can trust your body's current capabilities, yoga can become a means to lose weight fast.

A Powerful Exception

One form of yoga which *can* help you lose weight, according to many experts and physical trainers, is called Vinyasa yoga. It involves a series of 'sun salutations,' with various postures, done without any breaks in between. The postures are usually very challenging, and become progressively harder over the course of the session. You're also expected to breathe normally while doing Vinyasa yoga.

Vinyasa raises your heart rate and keeps it at an elevated rate throughout the session, which is what will eventually help you lose weight. But practicing any form of Vinyasa yoga requires a reasonable level of fitness, and beginners will need to improve their flexibility and strength before they get to that level. The most popular form of Vinyasa yoga, especially in the West, is Power Yoga. Power Yoga has now become a generic term, used for any strenuous and intense yoga session, and is practiced in many different ways.

Indirect Weight Loss Benefits of Yoga

Apart from directly burning calories to help you shed excess weight, yoga has several indirect weight loss benefits. First, it tones and strengthens your muscles, improving your metabolic rate to burn more calories while at rest. And, by reducing your stress levels, improving your sense of well-being, and making you connect with and understand your body better, it helps control and regulate your appetite, making you less prone to overeating. This is why yoga is so effective for people who are already at a near-perfect weight and want to keep those excess pounds off.

Yoga offers more than just burning calories. It gives you a complete health package, promotes good habits, and improves your base of strength and flexibility. So, whatever other weight loss exercises you take up, you'll be able to do them productively, enjoy them, and protect yourself from injuries.

78

A Balanced Diet for Vegans and Vegetarians to Lose Weight Fast

If you've been busy looking for tips on how to lose weight fast, you know by now there are no magic secrets out there. Weight loss supplements aren't effective without a healthy lifestyle, and drastic, restrictive fad diets are detrimental to long-term health and weight loss plans. There's no substitute for a healthy and balanced diet. The good news is that, even if you're a vegetarian or vegan, you'll find all the nutrients your body needs in nature.

Proteins

One major concern for vegetarians and vegans is getting enough protein. Yes, meat eaters end up eating more proteins than vegans and vegetarians, but they're actually eating protein in excess of what the human body needs. For vegetarians, milk and milk products are a great source of protein, and a vital source of calcium and vitamin B12. Beans, lentils, seeds, nuts and grains also contain substantial amounts of protein for both vegetarians and vegans. Even some vegetables, such as corn, count as important sources of protein.

Iron and Zinc

It's easier for the body to absorb iron and zinc from animal products than from plant foods, so vegetarians and vegans need to be particularly conscious of eating foods rich in these nutrients. Iron is found in peas, leafy green vegetables, cooked dried beans, lentils, and iron-fortified grain products. Zinc is also available from lentil and dried beans, but also from soy, whole-grain bread, and several kinds of vegetables.

Omega-3 Fatty Acids

The best source for vital omega-3 fatty acids are fish and eggs, but vegans and vegetarians can get this nutrient from leafy greens, hemp, pumpkin, and flax seeds, walnuts, canola oil, and soya bean oil.

Calcium

As we mentioned, lacto-vegetarians don't need to worry about calcium deficiencies, but neither do vegans, provided their diet is rich in leafy green vegetables, soy products, broccoli and beans. Fortified fruit juices also contain calcium, but watch the calories and sugar! Vitamin B12 is the only nutrient vegans won't find in their diet, so they should take a supplement for this. They also risk vitamin D deficiency; they can either take a supplement, or spend time in the sun. Fifteen minutes of unprotected exposure to sunlight per day is all you need, however; any more than that, and be sure to apply sunscreen.

Vegetarians and vegans can lose weight fast *and* enjoy great health, provided they follow a varied diet of healthy recipes. The great advantage of being a vegetarian is that vegetables—and all their vital nutrients—probably already figure into your diet in a big way. If they don't, try incorporating them into your diet in interesting ways—try making them more a part of your main course, instead of just as a side dish.

79

How to Lose Weight Fast During the Holiday Season

Winter is when people are generally keenest to learn tips on how to lose weight fast. It's not surprising, since the body has a tendency to store fat during the winter months. And Christmas and New Years are just around the corner, with parties, feasts, pies, sweet treats and alcohol in abundance. In these circumstances, it might seem impossible to get slim and keep those excess pounds off. It's certainly not impossible, though—just follow these simple weight loss tips.

Exercise is Invaluable

You don't have to force yourself out into the bitter cold just for a workout, when you could go down to the gym and warm up on the treadmill or stationary bike. If it's so bitterly cold you can't even consider leaving your house, there are a host of exercises you can do in your own living room, like Pilates, yoga, jump rope, and body-weight resistance exercises. Just thirty minutes a day will help you lose weight.

Resisting Christmas Temptations

Temptation is everywhere you turn during the holiday season, but you don't need to deny yourself every treat. Besides, sitting in the corner with your salad and watching everyone else enjoy their cookies is depressing, and can cause a negative mindset. So, go ahead and enjoy your Christmas. Just control your intake of sweets, sodas, high-calorie and junk foods in the weeks leading up to Christmas. A day or two of indulgence won't cause any lasting harm, but a few weeks can really cripple your weight loss efforts.

Alcohol

Alcohol is probably the worst culprit of weight gain, especially during the holidays. Most people don't realize that a glass of red wine has 120 calories; a pint of beer has 180. Try to avoid alcohol as much as you can during the holiday season. If you must imbibe, try to make one drink last, instead of having several drinks.

Drink Enough Water

Water is a highly-underrated weight loss tool. Most people don't drink enough water to begin with, but especially during winter, which slows down their metabolism, and can lead to the body misinterpreting thirst as hunger. Try to have a full glass of water half an hour before a meal, and you'll likely end up eating less.

A Healthy Breakfast

A healthy breakfast gives your metabolism a morning jumpstart, and prevents you from overeating throughout the rest of the day. The healthiest options are boiled eggs, fruit, a sandwich with low-calorie dressing and lean meat like chicken or fish on whole wheat bread, or even whole-grain cereal with skim milk.

It's best to begin your weight loss effort at least a few weeks before Christmas. That'll give you time to lose a few pounds, so even if you splurge during Christmas and New Year's, the damage won't be too serious. But be sure to approach your weight loss journey with a positive attitude. Believe in your capability to lose weight, and be patient—don't expect miracles.

80

I Want to Lose Weight Fast, but Not by Following Ridiculous Diet Fads

"**I** want to lose weight!" "I want to get slim!" "I want a figure like such-and-such celebrity!" These are the cries heard round the world by an overwhelming number of people. Under pressure from the media, their peers, and their own self-image, it's not uncommon for them to fall victim to a "diet program" (read: *fad*) endorsed by one celebrity or another.

But what most people don't stop to think about is how these celebrities can have any form of nutritional training. Most are swayed by their good looks and figure; that seems to be proof enough of their credibility. Surely, if they look like that, the diet must work?

But a great figure doesn't mean great nutrition and health. Celebrities are *celebrities*; they're not nutritionists, physical trainers, or doctors. They have no special knowledge of nutrition, physiology, muscle building, or holistic weight loss. There are many factors to weight loss that only an expert can fully account for.

Nutrition experts will tell you that most of these diet fads endorsed by celebrities are based on fiction and half-baked truths. Some will assist in weight loss, sure, but the moment you return to your normal diet, your weight will return, too, possibly with interest.

Take the Cabbage Soup Diet. It's simple; you survive on a diet of as much cabbage soup as you can stomach. Not only is this fad diet ridiculous, impractical, and unappetizing, it can also be quite dangerous. To begin with, it hasn't been endorsed by any of the leading health organizations; in fact, the American Heart Association has actually disavowed this diet, saying it does more harm than good.

Does cabbage soup help you lose weight? Yes, but most of your weight loss will be water weight, not fat. The Cabbage Soup Diet also has several uncomfortable and potentially dangerous side effects, like stomach pains, weakness, and diarrhea.

We're not making a blanket dismissal of every diet plan out there. But if you feel you need the guidance of a super-structured diet, then go for a plan formulated by a diet specialist, a professional trainer, or a nutritional expert. In other words, trust people who know what they're talking about, not those who capitalize on their celebrity status and great figure (which is more likely the result of genetic good luck than cabbage soup!) to manipulate you, and don't allow yourself to be taken for a ride by people who are being paid to sell you diet fads.

So, the next time you cry "I want to lose weight!" add "Sensibly and intelligently!" at the end of the sentence. That's not just the right way; it's the only way.

81

Eat Your Veggies to Lose Weight Fast and Easy – 5 Simple Facts

If you want to lose weight fast and keep your body slim and healthy, it's the simple things you do that matter, like incorporating more vegetables into your diet. Most people have heard this advice so often, dating back to their childhood, that they just don't pay attention anymore. But if you focus your attention for just a moment, you'll learn how eating a variety of vegetables is an essential ingredient of any weight loss plan.

How Vegetables Help You Lose Weight

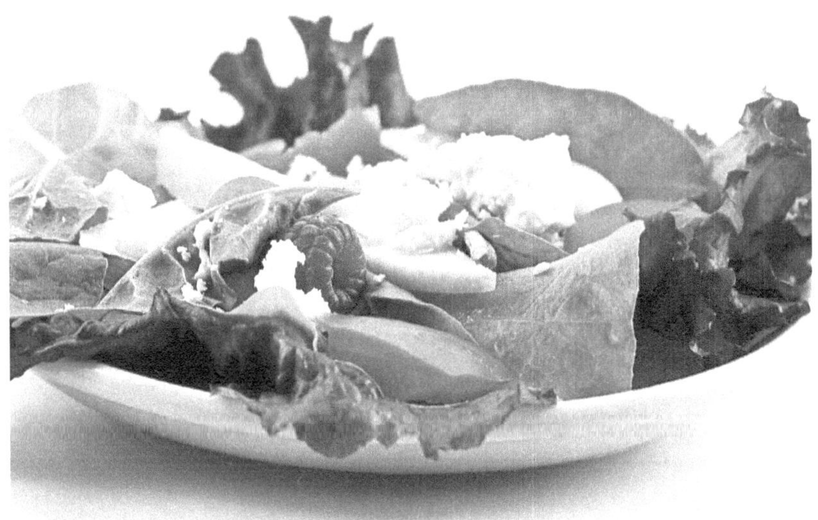

Nearly all vegetables are high in fiber and low in calories. Combined with their excellent nutritive value and health benefits, you have an unbeatable combination for a weight loss diet. How it works is simple: all the fiber in vegetables make the digestive system work harder to break down the food, meaning the body has to burn more calories during digestion than it would on, say, a burger and fries. And while your body is burning more calories breaking down all those vegetables, you'll actually be eating less. Vegetables might have a lower calorie-to-mass ratio than other foods, but their fiber-to-mass ratio is high, leaving you pleasantly full until your next mealtime.

The Two Kinds

There are two kinds of vegetables: starchy and non-starchy. The non-starchy ones are what you should be eating more of, because they're low in sugar. Starchy vegetables are just the opposite. Except for potatoes, corn, peas, squash, plantains and yams, all other common vegetables are non-starchy. That doesn't mean avoid starchy vegetables altogether—they're still vegetables, after all, and have great nutritional value—but consume them in much more careful moderation than non-starchy vegetables.

Recommended Portions

The USDA (United States Department of Agriculture) recommends three or more cups of vegetables a day for a healthy adult, only half a cup of which should be starchy vegetables.

Free Foods

Some vegetables are so low in calories they're known as 'free foods.' These include carrots, mushrooms, cauliflower, radishes, cucumbers, fresh green beans, cabbage, cherry tomatoes, lettuce, and celery. 'Free foods' are foods you can eat unlimited quantities of, without worrying about calorie counts. Just be careful not to drench your 'free foods' in fatty dressings or dips, or you'll undo all their benefits.

Nutrient-Rich

Apart from their weight-loss benefits, vegetables are super-rich in nutrients, like vitamins, minerals, and phytochemicals. Ideally, one should have a variety of vegetables, instead of sticking to one or two types, since each vegetable has its own unique balance of these nutrients. One easy rule of thumb is to try and eat as much *color* as possible; this will ensure you're getting a healthy balance of vitamins and minerals. For maximum benefits, vegetables are best eaten raw, baked, or steamed. If they're boiled and eaten without their stalk, most of the nutrients go into the trash with the stalk.

If you're trying to eat more vegetables to lose weight fast, but find you're having to force yourself, change your strategy. Instead of putting veggies on the side or munching a raw salad, try incorporating more vegetables into your main dish itself. Eggplant makes a great substitute for lasagna noodles, for example, and you can substitute spiralized zucchini for pasta. Cauliflower can be riced for risotto, or you can even make a great pizza crust from it! You're not the only one who struggles to eat their vegetables; a little research will net plenty of recipes from people who've faced this problem themselves and conquered it with a little ingenuity.

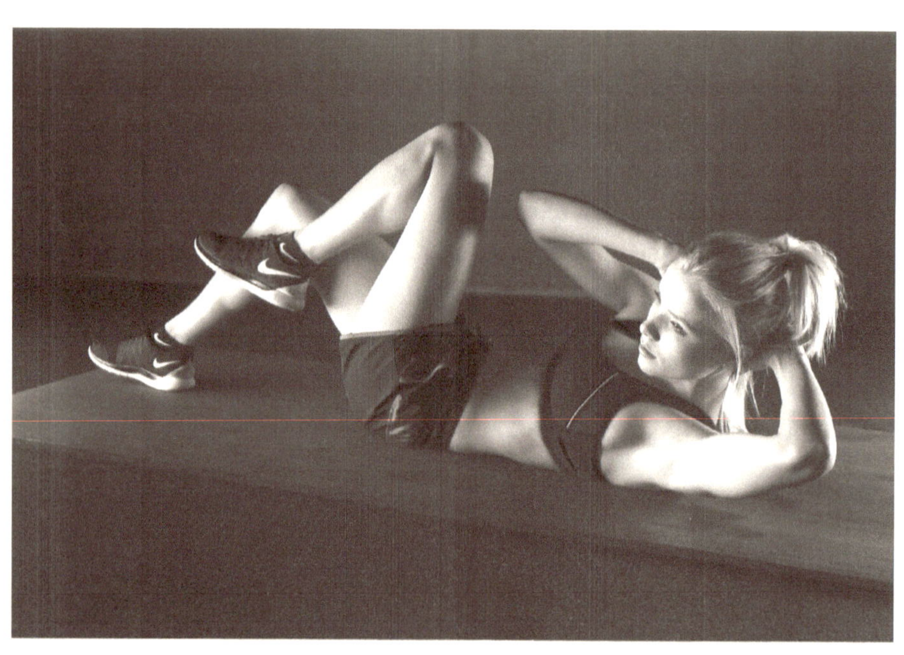

82

How to Get a Butt Like Jennifer Lopez – Follow These 5 Mind Boggling Tips

Let's face it—Jennifer Lopez has the sexiest butt on this planet. It drives guys crazy with desire and makes girls go green with envy. So how can you get a butt like JLo? Well, it won't be a piece of cake; there's some hard work involved, but the compliments will make it all worthwhile. Here are some exercises to get that shapely, killer butt:

Squats

Squats are some of the best exercises to get your butt in shape. Stand with your feet slightly wider than hip-width apart. Keeping your back straight, tighten your abs, and squat, being careful to keep your knees behind your toes. When you return to standing, squeeze your butt muscles as though you were trying to hold back gas. Do two to three sets of eight to twelve reps each. If you want to increase the intensity once you've perfected your form, you can add weights.

Lunges

There are several types of lunges: the classic front lunge, wheel lunges, side-to-side lunges, walking lunges, and reverse lunges. All of the types can be pretty challenging, since they work various muscle groups simultaneously, including the glutes, hamstrings, quads, and calves. Again, once you've perfected the form, you can take this exercise to the next level by raising your back foot on a platform or step.

Hip Extension

Hip extensions, also known as donkey kicks, work on the largest muscle group of the body, the gluteus maximus. Get down on all fours, with your hands directly under your shoulders and your knees directly under your hips. Keeping your knee bent at a ninety degree angle, swing one leg straight back behind you, so the sole of your foot points straight at the ceiling, and squeeze your glutes at the top. If you're looking for additional challenge, place a dumbbell behind your knee, or use ankle weights to increase the intensity. For an interesting variation, lie down with your torso and hips supported by an exercise ball. Place your hands on the floor, bend your knees, squeeze your glutes and point your feet straight up at the ceiling.

Leg Raises

Lie down flat on your back, with a towel under your hips if you're on a hard floor. Inhale, and lift your legs so they form a 90 degree angle to your body. Exhale, and lower your legs toward the floor without letting them touch. Keep your legs floating an inch or two off the ground for a count of ten, then raise them back up. Do two to three sets of ten reps each.

Cardiovascular Exercises

You should also incorporate a variety of cardiovascular exercises in your workout routine. Swimming, jogging, riding a stationary or traditional bike, or walking briskly are excellent cardiovascular exercises. Jogging and cycling in particular will help tone your butt while sweating out the calories. Cycling can be even more effective if you stand up to pedal, instead of sitting down.

83

The Best Way to Lose Weight Fast – Go Fruity!

Years of research and thousands of supplements and theories later, science has finally validated your Grandma's advice. It turns out that eating a healthy amount of fruit is one of the most crucial strategies to lose weight fast. What's more, fruits offer you a multitude of other health benefits, apart from weight loss. In other words, eating fruit should be at the top of your list of permanent, healthy lifestyle changes.

The Weight Loss Advantages of Fruits

There are two simple reasons why fruits help you lose weight. First, they're low in calories, so every time you swap a bar of chocolate for a piece of fruit, you end up consuming far fewer calories. Second, fruits are high in fiber, which means they'll leave you feeling far fuller than that chocolate bar would have, saving you from the temptation of bingeing on unhealthy goodies. And third, fruit offers sustained energy, instead of the sugar spike and subsequent crash junk food will give you.

The Ideal Amount

Ideally, you should try to eat five portions of fruit daily. To put that into real-world terms, that would be four to five plums, a medium bunch of grapes, and two bananas. Eating a large fruit like a melon counts as two to three servings. If you find five portions a day too inconvenient or expensive, eat whatever amount is feasible for you. Something is always better than nothing!

The Need for Variety

Rather than just eating five bananas every day, try to mix it up. Fruits are rich in vitamins, minerals and phytochemicals, all of which exist in varying amounts in different fruits. Color is the primary indicator of these ratios, so mix up your colors, and you'll end up with a healthy nutrient balance.

Encouraging Yourself

Try different techniques to incorporate fruit into your diet. Add fresh or dried fruit to your breakfast cereal, put a piece of fruit in your purse or briefcase as you head off to work, try unsweetened juices, place your fruit bowl next to your TV, or even prepare a large bowl of fruit salad and store it in your fridge. Very soon, you may find yourself addicted to this healthy habit!

Finally, bear in mind that simply eating fruit is not enough to lose weight fast, if your other habits aren't healthy. What you need is an all-around balanced diet, of which fruit is a crucial part, and exercise is also essential to achieve your weight loss goals.

84

How to Lose Face Fat Fast and Easy – 5 Mind Blowing Tips to Get a Sculpted Face

The first thing people see when they look at you is your face. A well-toned face, without sagging muscles or double chins, is a sight that gets attention. A face that's puffy and bloated can get attention, too, but for the wrong reasons.

When we talk about a well-toned face, don't think we're referring to an emaciated visage, with eyes popping in their sockets. That's hardly anyone's definition of beauty. But if you want a smooth, healthy-looking face, here are a few tips to help you.

1. Cut Refined Carbs & Sugar

Too many carbohydrates, such as white flour, cause the body to retain water, especially in the hands, ankles, and face. Dropping simple carbs from your diet and switching to whole grains like oatmeal can result in a drastic change in your water retention, and you'll notice a reduction in facial puffiness after a few days. The change is great for your overall fitness, as well.

2. Go Easy on the Salt

Excess salt can cause water retention in the same areas. Cut back on foods like chips and canned soups, which often contain unhealthy amounts of sodium. Salt tastes great on the palate, but it's bound to show up in your face later.

3. Water, Water, Water

Contrary to popular belief, water retention isn't caused by drinking a lot of water; in fact, it's quite the opposite. When you drink enough water, the body stops storing it in unsightly places. So make sure you drink at least eight glasses of water a day, and you'll see a difference in not only your face's puffiness, but also the quality of your skin.

4. Check your Medication

If you're on any kind of prescription or over-the-counter medications, check to see if they list water retention as a side effect. If so, speak to your physician about alternatives—but don't, under any circumstances, discontinue your medication without consulting your physician first.

5. Do Facial Exercises

There are a range of facial exercises which can help you lose facial fat and tone your muscle structure. They can help slim down your double chin, reduce the chubbiness of your cheeks, and give you a slim, firm overall look. These exercises help tighten and lift the muscles of your face, in addition to burning fat in those problem areas. These exercises can be found easily on the internet and hardly take more than a few minutes to do. You'll see results in just a few weeks.

85

How to Lose Weight Fast and Easy – 10 Great Tips to Help You Lose Weight Quickly

We're not sure how it was in the past, but today, society is obsessed with weight loss and achieving a slim, trim figure. Man, in his vanity, wants nothing less than perfection for himself and those around him. Overweight people suffer from a lot more than just health problems; their self-confidence is under constant attack, leading to severe depression in many cases. It's no wonder people want to lose weight quickly and easily in order to feel better about themselves. The ideas below can help you lose weight and get slim, and they might end up changing your whole life for the better.

- If you feel thirsty, water is your best friend, and carbonated drinks or even sugary juices are your enemy. Nothing can replace water's function in the body, so make sure you drink at least eight glasses a day.

- Trash the convention of three meals a day. Stuffing your body with food in a single sitting does it no good; break the same amount of food up into five or six smaller meals or healthy snacks per day. This keeps your metabolism on its toes, and helps the body release less insulin which, in turn, keeps blood sugar levels steady and controls hunger pangs.

- Keep plenty of low-fat yogurt in the fridge, and have it three times a day. You can cut down on almost 500 calories a day this way. Do this for twelve weeks, and watch the weight come off!

- For breakfast, have a serving of whole-grain cereal five days a week. This gives your body plenty of calcium, and helps you stay full for longer.

- Learn to distinguish between false and real hunger pangs. If you feel hungry, drink a glass of water and wait a while before eating. False hunger pangs usually pass in a few minutes, saving you from putting unnecessary calories in your body.

- If you enjoy dressing on your salad or sauces on your food, opt for flavorings like salsa, Cajun seasonings, and hot sauce in place of creamy, sugary, or buttery sauces. They have fewer calories, and are delicious, too!

- Instead of drinking fruit juices, have the fruit. It will keep you satisfied for longer, and you'll have fewer calories to deal with, too.

- Make it a habit to walk regularly, especially if you can't make time for exercise. Walk to the grocery store, or get off the bus or subway earlier and walk the rest of the way. These tiny modifications have big results, as you'll soon see.

- Once a week, manually deep-clean something in the house. Scrub the floors, wash the windows, clean the bathroom tiles. Your house will sparkle, and you'll burn four calories a minute!

- Go for a walk before dinner. Not only does it help burn calories, it also curbs your appetite.

86

5 Golden Rules to Exercise for Fast and Easy Weight Loss

I f you're looking to lose weight fast, and improve your overall health and wellbeing in the process, there's nothing more beneficial or advisable than regular exercise. Most of the 'flab to fab' stories don't just involve weight loss pills, supplements, or diets, as ads would have you believe. Some form of exercise is invariably involved in losing weight and gaining good health.

The Kinds of Exercises

An effective weekly exercise routine should consist of three kinds of exercise: cardiovascular, such as brisk walking, jogging, or cycling; muscle-building and strengthening, which usually involves some form of weight training; and stretching and flexibility. Each offers their own set of advantages for someone who wants to lose weight. Cardiovascular exercises increase your heart rate while you're exercising, burning excess calories in the process. Muscle-building and strengthening exercises improve your BMR, or the rate at which your body burns calories, since muscles need far more energy than fat. Stretching and flexibility improve posture and range of motion, helping protect you from injury.

20 Minutes of Cardio

As far as cardiovascular exercises go, to burn a significant amount of calories, you need to keep at it for a spell of at least twenty minutes. Short bursts of exercise aren't as effective for slimming down as a longer, continuous spell. If you haven't exercised for a long time, start with a brisk walk for twenty to thirty minutes, and then you can gradually replace it with a jog over the next several weeks.

The Right Way to Begin

If you haven't been physically active for a few years, it's best to begin by consulting a physician to discuss which exercises are most suitable for you.

Variety Is the Key

The good news is the human body adapts very quickly. That's also the bad news. You'll see yourself getting stronger and faster every day, but once your body adapts to a routine, it'll be able to complete it with less effort. That means you'll be burning fewer calories during the exact same workout, and your muscle development will stagnate. Once this happens, your exercise won't lead to further weight loss. The key is variety, and putting your body through new and higher levels of challenge.

Give Yourself a Break!

The period of rest following an exercise routine is just as important as the exercise itself, because this is when muscles repair, grow, and become stronger. So if you're overenthusiastic and don't give yourself enough recovery time, you won't be getting strong, toned muscles and faster weight loss—you'll be risking fatigue, burnout, and injury. Beginners should allow themselves two to three days of *complete* rest from serious exercise every week.

If you want to lose weight fast with some exercise, it's not necessary to wait around until you find time to hit the gym. Simply adopting a more active general lifestyle will start you off on your weight loss goals. Taking the stairs instead of the elevator, even if it's just a flight or two, and if you have to go a short distance, walk briskly instead of pulling out your car. You can even pick up a sport you enjoy on the weekends.

87

Your Master Key to Fast Weight Loss – Exercise as You Go

One universal difficulty of today's world is that there's simply no time to accommodate an exercise routine. With such sedentary lifestyles, how can we hope to achieve weight loss? And even putting the concern of weight loss aside, we don't even have time to keep our bodies fit and healthy.

Exercise is very important—no one can argue that. However, it's also true that most people have such hectic lifestyles that they can't make time to go to a gym or have a proper workout routine. There's way too much on our plates already, isn't there?

1. Pumping Iron Isn't the Only Form of Exercise

Having said that, we'll also point out that exercise can be more than lifting weight in the gym, running laps on a track, or spending money on expensive fitness centers. Exercise means keeping yourself active and your body in momentum. If you look around, there are plenty of things you can do to add a little bit of exercise into the most fast-paced routine. They may not lead to drastic weight loss, but you'll be stronger and have a healthier life overall.

2. Approach Your Workout with Intelligence

Let's clear up another misconception—you don't need to exercise for forty-five minutes or an hour to lose weight. If you don't have that kind of time, a better option would be to break up your exercise routine into shorter, more manageable sessions, so you have multiple workouts in one day, instead of doing nothing at all. This way, there's less pressure for you to make time for a workout. Even better, research has shown those who do shorter bouts of exercise find it easier to stick to their routine. They exercise more days per week, and achieve more weight loss than those who exercise for an extended period of time in a day.

3. Intelligent Workouts Tips for Busy Bees

Here are some tips that don't require you to make any major changes in your life, and yet will help you stay slim and get fit:

- Skip the elevator; use the stairs.

- If your office is relatively close to home, walk or bike to work. You'll burn calories, lose weight, and save money on gas.

- If you take the bus or subway to work, get off a stop earlier and walk the rest of the way.

- Keep light weights handy around your cubicle, and sneak a quick workout session in during lunch or coffee breaks. If your office has an in-house fitness center, even better! Make time for short ten-minute workouts twice a day.

88

Want to Lose Weight Fast? Beware of 4 Common Myths That Can Sabotage Your Dreams

There are a lot of weight loss myths out there. In spite of living proudly in the 'information age,' people are still full of misinformation about how to lose weight quickly, healthily, and consistently.

Myth 1: I Can Worry About All-around Fat Loss Later; First, Let Me Get Rid of This Weight Around My Belly

This is the thought process that drives people to buy sauna belts and other 'belly fat' gadgets of the 'As Seen On TV!' variety. The truth is that there's no known way to get rid of belly fat specifically without also getting rid of thigh, face, or arm fat. Fat loss is not a process that can be targeted to certain areas; it's an all-or-nothing proposition, and with the right diet and exercise, one can start burning body fat. Sauna belts never gave anyone a body to die for; all they do is drain the water out from around your waist in the form of sweat. As soon as you replenish that water, it all goes right back where it started!

Myth 2: the Best Way to Lose Weight Rapidly is That Miraculous Two-week Diet I Heard About

Any extremely low-calorie, drastic, and unbalanced diet that puts your body through extreme self-denial is hazardous to your health and, incidentally, counter-productive to your weight loss goals. Sure, in the short run there's no faster way to shed pounds than a 'crash' diet, but such a diet truly is like a crash for your body; it sends it into shock, and in order to deal with the famine conditions, slows your metabolism down dramatically. As soon as you return to a normal diet, your metabolism won't even be able to burn a maintenance amount of calories, and all that weight will pile right back on.

Myth 3: to Lose Weight, I Must Eat Less

Surprisingly, overweight people aren't always overeaters. The key to weight loss is not necessarily eating less, but eating healthier. By starving yourself, you'll do the same thing to your body as a crash diet does, with the exact same results. What you should be trying to do instead is cut the calorie-rich fats and artificial sugars from your diet, and replacing them with healthier alternatives. A wholesome and balanced diet speeds up your metabolism and reduces your calorie intake—the two most desirable conditions for weight loss. And rather than having two or three large meals a day, have four or five smaller meals. That's right, eat more often to lose weight. By making your body digest food more frequently, you'll be burning calories and speeding up your metabolism.

Myth 4: If I Want to Get Slim, I Better Start Going for a Jog

A cardiovascular exercise such as jogging will help you burn a fair amount of calories, it's true, but at the end of the day—literally—it's not as effective as muscle-building. Muscle training not only burns calories during exercise, but also when you're sitting quietly at your desk, or fast asleep at night. Muscles need constant fuel, even while your body's at rest. The more muscles you have, the more calories you burn overall, and the faster you'll achieve your goals.

89

Do Your Cardio Right and Lose Weight Fast

Traditionally, people have associated weight loss and better health with cardiovascular exercises such as brisk walking, jogging, running or cycling. They're not wrong, but people tend to settle down into a routine they insist on practicing every day, such as a thirty-minute jog. That's where things go wrong. Here's the right way to do cardiovascular exercises in order to lose weight fast:

Strategy 1: Interval Training

The human body is amazingly adaptable. If you subject it to a routine for a long enough period, it will become very efficient at it, needing less and less effort to complete it. What this means is that you're no longer burning enough calories on your daily jog to spur your fitness; as a result, you may have stagnated in your weight loss, too. What you need is to discard your routine, and discover the amazing benefits of interval training.

Faster Weight Loss in Less Time

It sounds complex, but interval training is very simple. It refers to any cardiovascular exercise where short, intense bursts of fast activity are alternated with periods of light intensity or rest. So, if you punctuate your run with thirty seconds of sprinting every two minutes, that's interval training. Do eight sets of two minutes of jogging and thirty seconds of running, and in just twenty minutes you'll have spurred your metabolism and fitness a lot more than your usual jog. The direct result is faster weight loss. According to a study, if people who do light intensity, long-duration cardiovascular workouts switch to interval training, they can achieve their weight loss goals by cutting their total exercise time to less than half.

Interval training 101

Interval training may involve either an increase in speed/intensity or an increase in resistance for a pre-set duration, and can be done with any cardiovascular exercise, whether it's running, jumping rope, cycling or swimming, and can involve dozens of variations. On the whole, it's far less monotonous and more enjoyable than low-intensity, consistent cardio, and prevents the body from adapting and subsequently stagnating. As your fitness improves, you can make your intervals longer or more challenging, and reduce the period of rest and recovery between intervals. Even twenty minutes of interval training, three to four times a week, will end up being incomparably more effective for fast weight loss than a consistent daily effort.

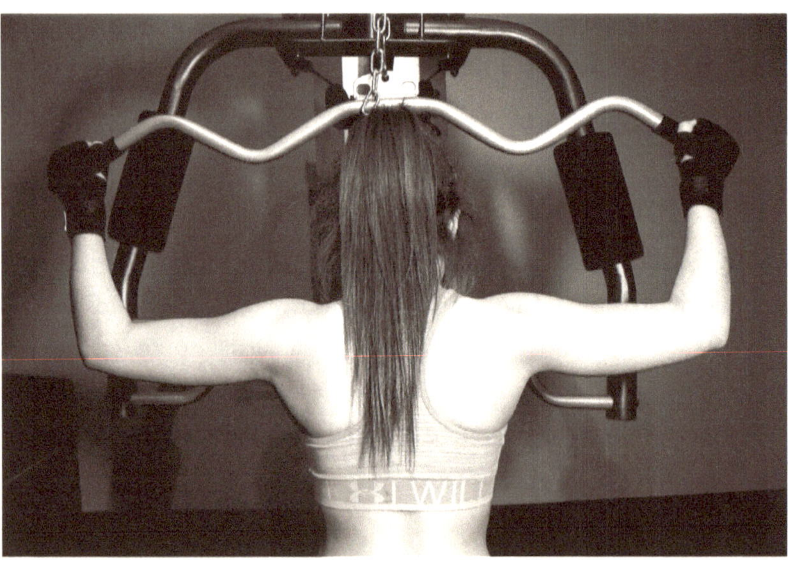

Strategy 2: Varying your Exercise

Apart from interval training, another strategy to spur your fitness and get slim faster is to vary your cardiovascular exercise itself. If you're running or jogging 5 days a week, try and replace it with cycling or swimming for one or two days. This will engage and develop new muscle groups, and your metabolism will get a boost, which of course directly translates to faster weight loss. And, since the exercise is new and more challenging, your body will burn more calories during the workout itself. All it takes is a few weeks, and you'll be smiling at the mirror!

90

Detoxify Your Body, Speed Up Your Metabolism and Lose Weight Fast!

Everyone wants to lose weight fast. You should know by now that we don't believe in overnight weight loss or miraculous inch reduction in a week's time, but we do know that, if you follow certain tips, you can speed up the process of weight loss a bit. Here, we provide tips on how to detoxify your body and increase your metabolism.

Detox your Body Naturally

It's important to detoxify your body regularly to help it work at peak capacity. Once your organs are working more efficiently, they'll aid in your body's overall fitness and health. The good news is you can detox easily and naturally with the following foods:

- **Strawberries and Cherries:** These fruits are rich sources of ellagic acid, a nutrient which helps fight toxins and pollutants in the body, and gets rid of free radicals.

- **Grapes:** Grapes are a cornucopia of flavinols, which help the blood run smoothly through the body and keep the arteries working in mint condition.

- **Citrus fruits:** All citrus fruits are great sources of vitamins C and E, which cleanse the liver and keep it working efficiently.

- **Prunes:** Prunes are known for their colon-cleansing properties. In addition, they also stimulate the gut to help the body rid itself of waste.

- **Apricots:** Apricots are rich in vitamin C and beta carotene. Smokers and former smokers in particular will benefit from eating apricots, since it repairs damage to the lungs caused by smoking.

- **Cranberries:** Cranberries contain proanthocyanidin. This antioxidant cleanses the kidneys and flushes out toxins.

Increase your Metabolism

Now that you've detoxified your body, it's time to boost your metabolism, so your body can burn stored fats faster, and help you lose weight more quickly.

Drink Ice Water: While this suggestion might not be great for your throat, drinking ice water causes the body to burn up to a hundred calories, since it needs to heat the water and bring it to body temperature.

Green Tea: Research has proven that having green tea five times a day can burn up to eighty calories, just like that! The antioxidants present in green tea are known to boost your body's metabolism.

Mustard and Chili Sauce: If you're not averse to hot and spicy foods, mustard and chili sauce can boost your body's calorie-burning capacity by five to ten percent. These foods contain capsaicin, a compound which speeds up your metabolism.

Low-Fat Dairy: Low-fat dairy foods are a great source of calcium. While breaking down and processing the calcium, the body is forced to use fat from its cells, thereby burning stored fat in the body. In addition, low-fat dairy products also reduce the amount of fat absorbed by the body. Not only do they help you lose weight fast, but they can also keep it from coming back.

91

The Essential Tips to Lose Weight Fast

Weight loss isn't rocket science. There are no 'secret strategies,' so you have no reason to feel daunted. All it takes is a few healthy changes to your lifestyle, and maintaining that lifestyle permanently.

Increasing your Metabolism is Key

It's important to understand that weight is about more than just cutting calories. In fact, many overweight people don't actually overeat, and don't need to cut their overall calorie consumption. Rather, the key to weight loss is increasing the rate at which your body burns calories, i.e. your metabolism.

Drink Lots of Water to Get Slim!

This is the easiest lifestyle change to incorporate, and also the most neglected. Most people don't drink enough water, even though water is the most natural, healthiest drink for human beings. You should be drinking at least eight to ten glasses of water per day; this will help cleanse your system of toxins as well as boost your metabolism. And, if you substitute water for those sugary glasses of cola and iced tea, you'll automatically be cutting down on empty calories. If you feel like something sweet, try unsweetened juice instead of soda.

Cut Down on Processed Foods

Processed foods, fried foods, sugary meals and refined flour-based recipes not only load your body with unhealthy and unnecessary calories, they also slow your metabolism. Replace these with wholesome, natural and unprocessed meals as much as possible. At *least* one portion of fruits and vegetables per day is a must. If you're feeling peckish between meals, have some fruit rather than chips or chocolate.

Lean Proteins

Your meals, breakfast in particular, should include a source of lean protein. Lean proteins make you feel satisfied, boost your metabolism, and keep your insulin and blood sugar levels regulated. Seeds, nuts, chicken, fish and eggs are the best natural sources of lean protein.

Eat Frequently

Many people think starving themselves is the way to lose weight. After all, whoever heard of a diet where you eat *more* instead of less? But that's exactly what you should be doing. If you don't eat frequently, your body prepares for long-term starvation by storing fat instead of burning it. Eating small, frequent meals at least five to six times daily reassures your body that food is abundant, so it doesn't feel the need to store extra energy in the form of fat. Not only that, but every time your body digests food, it burns calories, so the more often you engage it in digestion, the faster your metabolism. And all you're doing is eating smarter, not more—if you're aiming for 2000 calories per day, you'll split that amount up into five meals, rather than three.

Exercise

Finally, you have to remember that diet is only half the battle. Exercise is just as important. Try to incorporate some cardiovascular exercise into your routine. For instance, start your day with a twenty minute brisk walk before breakfast. If you like more of a challenge, you can try running, swimming, cycling, or, really, any sport that gets you moving. Just make sure that, whatever exercise you choose, do it for at least twenty minutes to reap the full health benefits.

92

A Low-Fat Diet to Lose Weight Fast

It's no revelation that foods high in fats are also packed with calories, and, if you want to lose weight fast, these are the kinds of foods you need to avoid. It's a well-known general principle that weight loss involves burning more calories than you consume, and that principle is best applied with a low-fat diet.

Going Low-Fat and Healthy

Before starting a low-fat diet, it's important to know a few things. First, just because a food item has less fat, that doesn't necessarily mean it's healthy. Sugar, for instance, has little fat, but it's packed with calories, and a diet high in sugar can spell disaster for someone looking to lose or maintain their weight. The best strategy is to choose low-fat foods with good overall nutritional value and low calorie density.

Second, not all fats are bad. Some fat is essential for the body, such as healthy omega-3 and unsaturated fats, which help control cholesterol levels and prevent heart disease. As a rule of thumb, thirty percent of your entire calorie consumption should be from fats, and most of those fat calories should be from the healthy fats mentioned above. Omega-3 is found in some varieties of fish, such as salmon, fresh tuna, and sardines, as well as certain vegetable oils and plant foods. Unsaturated fats are mainly found in healthy vegetable oils like rapeseed, olive, corn and sunflower oil, as well as various nuts and fruits.

The Food Items to Avoid

Some of the popular food items to avoid while following a low-fat diet are whole milk, sweet goodies such as ice cream (unless it's low-fat!), chocolate, cake, cookies, chips, fried or roasted potatoes, coconut, pastries, croissants, white bread, refined-flour based pancakes and pastas, butter, duck meat, meat pies, and most cream and hard cheese. A typical pantry is full of at least some, if not all, of these food items, in the form of unhealthy snacks. If your kitchen is one of these, it might be a good idea to clean the shelves and replace these high-fat foods with healthy, fat-free ones.

Healthy, Low-Fat Food Items

A healthy diet with a moderate amount of fat should have plenty of variety and be practical enough to sustain for a long period of time. After all, your weight loss goals aren't just for the coming season! Some nutritious low-fat foods to replace all those fatty snacks are: skim milk, egg whites, low-fat yogurt, unsweetened fruit juice, chicken and fish, fresh and frozen vegetables and fruits, whole wheat breads, whole-grain pasta and rice, high fiber breakfast cereals, walnuts, baked potatoes, dried fruits, beans, legumes and pulses, and oatmeal. Even though it has a lot of variety, this isn't a complicated list, and most items on it can be readily and inexpensively found at your local grocery store. While the availability of healthy, low-fat foods might not be a problem, however, discipline will likely be the biggest challenge for those looking to lose weight fast.

It's important to keep in mind that weight loss isn't the only benefit of a diet plan based on these principles and food items. There are many associated health benefits, including higher energy levels, reduced risk of high cholesterol and heart problems, and even a reduced risk of cancer.

93

The Magic of the GI Tool to Lose Weight Fast

The subject of diet and nutrition is one which is constantly evolving and changing with new information, new trends and fads, and new studies. The latest buzz word is GI, or Glycemic Index. It's hit the public consciousness like a storm, and earned the attention of people looking to lose weight fast.

What is GI?

GI is an index which identifies the effect different food items have on blood sugar levels. Foods with high GI are those in which the carbohydrates are broken down quickly during digestion, leading to quick glucose release into the bloodstream. Low GI foods have carbohydrates which take a long time to break down, releasing glucose gradually into the system. The standard of measurement of GI is pure glucose, which has a GI of 100.

GI and Weight Loss

High-GI foods lead to a rapid increase in blood sugar levels, followed by a rapid drop. In terms of energy level, this means you'll experience a quick boost and an even more rapid crash, which can spell disaster for those with diabetes. That quick rise and drop in energy will also likely leave you feeling tired and hungry very soon after a high-GI meal, and you'll be tempted to pick up another snack. Low GI foods, on the other hand, take longer to break down and, with their consistent, gradual release of glucose, offer sustained energy for a longer period of time, leaving you satisfied for longer. So, naturally, people in the know who are trying to lose weight have begun gravitating toward low-GI foods.

Is GI a Perfect Indicator?

While the GI index is a good measure of foods which will tempt you to overeat, and those that will leave you satisfied longer, it's not a perfect yardstick for fast weight loss. If you're interested in slimming down, you can't rely solely on the GI. Some sugar-rich foods like ice cream and chocolate have a low GI, because of the high levels of fat and protein they contain, but obviously they're not healthy foods for those looking to lose weight quickly. Even adding oils, butter, or excessive salt to a meal can reduce its GI, but those certainly aren't healthy eating habits.

If you're trying to lose weight, the most important thing is to choose low-GI foods which have a high nutritional value, and to vary your diet so you're not missing any essential nutrients. Concentrating on one healthy, low GI food or food group isn't healthy.

The Healthy Low-GI Foods

Some healthy low-GI foods to help you lose weight fast are chicken, fish, eggs, legumes and pulses, whole grains, most fruits and vegetables, brown rice, oats, muesli, pasta, and bran. Don't make the mistake of giving up on medium- or high-GI foods—some of these, like skim milk, carrots, and watermelon carry significant health benefits.

94

I Want to Lose Weight Fast! – Okay, Get Your Facts Right First

When it comes to losing weight, most people are in a hurry, even though, deep down, they know shortcuts don't work. In their desperation to lose weight quickly, many people fall victim to half-baked truths and myths which have been passed down for generations.

If you want to lose weight, you have to begin by separating fact from fiction. Don't allow yourself to be guided by theories that can't be substantiated by science; it'll do you more harm than good, and slow, if not cripple, your weight loss efforts.

Myth #1: Carbohydrates Make You Fat

Carbohydrates are an essential part of a balanced diet; you simply cannot remove them completely to achieve weight loss. They're the fuel you need to run your body. Unless you have a moderate amount of carbs in your diet, you won't have the energy for day-to-day activities, much less a workout routine.

Do, however, swap simple carbohydrates, like soft drinks and sweets, in favor of complex carbohydrates like whole wheat bread, pasta, rice, and cereal, since these boost your body's metabolism and help you lose weight faster.

Myth #2: Avoid Fats at All Costs

Fats might be twice as fattening as carbs—it's right there in the name, after all—but that's no reason to cut them completely. Remember, any form of diet extreme isn't healthy; just as excess amounts of certain foods can be harmful, total deprivation can do just as much damage.

Studies have proven fats are required for a number of reasons. They protect the organs from shock, promote healthy function of the cells, maintain the temperature of the body, and have a host of other benefits. Can you imagine what would happen if you removed them from your diet completely?

Myth #3: Eating at Night Makes You Fat

Calories can't tell time! What matters is how many calories you consume in a day, not when you consume them. When a diet recommends you don't eat late, what they probably mean is not to have a full meal right before bed—that can give you indigestion. But there's no reason you can't have a light snack at night. It's certainly better for you than going to bed hungry

One final thought; the key to weight loss lies in moderation, not elimination. The body needs a balanced diet, and you can't throw out an entire food group without facing repercussions. Anyone who tells you that you need to starve yourself in order to lose weight is either trying to sell you something, or sadly misinformed. Eat healthy, avoid junk food, exercise regularly, and watch the weight drop in due course—the right way.

95

How to Lose Weight Quickly? Here is the Mantra to Lose Weight Fast and Easy

People are always looking for a secret that will help them lose weight quickly. But contrary to popular belief, there's nothing mysterious about successful weight loss programs. Making some healthy changes to your everyday life is a great way to drop those pounds quickly.

Eat!

Starving or fasting is *not* a prerequisite for any program to lose weight fast. While it's true that you need to reduce your calorie intake, you're not required to stop eating altogether. Just eat intelligently, and consume good carbs with a low glycemic index. For example, choose whole wheat bread over processed white bread, and brown rice as opposed to white rice. However, there is one important tenet of a weight loss diet—no junk food. There's no positive effect of eating junk food, so if you feel like snacking, snack healthy. Have a nutrition bar instead of a candy bar, and substitute low-fat cream for regular cream. When you feel the urge to binge, have fruits or salads instead.

One more thing—breakfast, lunch and dinner are a thing of the past. Professional trainers and nutritionists will now tell you it's far better to eat smaller meals spread throughout the day. This boosts your metabolism by keeping your body on its toes, and you stay fuller throughout the day and will be less inclined to snack.

Exercise and Keep Tabs

Regular exercise is mandatory—there's no way to avoid it. Do a combination of cardio, strength and endurance exercises, and aim for four to five thirty-minute sessions per week. And keep tabs on your exercise, through a fitness diary or tracking app. It'll make it easy to plan your exercise routine and work in the variety that will foil your ever-adapting body. If you did a session on the treadmill today, do some weightlifting tomorrow. At the end of the month, measure those inches to see how much you've achieved.

Those Small Changes We Talked About...

Still wondering how to lose weight fast? Just incorporate some basic changes into your life. Leave your car at home and walk or cycle to the office, if it's nearby. Take the stairs instead of the elevator, and during your breaks, try to get some exercise in your cubicle, like jumping jacks or running in place. Do some yoga, stretching, or calisthenics while you're watching TV and, if possible, get up early and go for a brisk walk around the park.

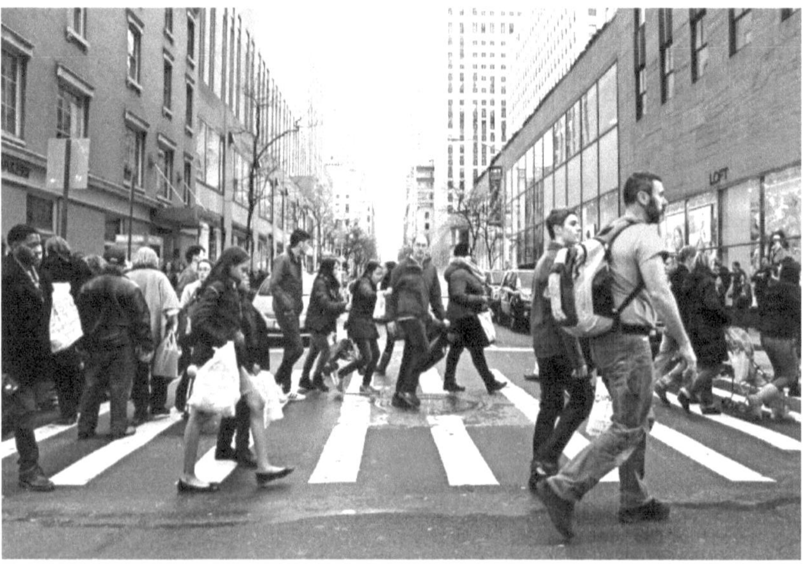

Conclusion

Stop looking for a magic mantra or fix to tell you how to lose weight quickly. There's no such thing, and you don't get anything in life from shortcuts. If you want to lose weight, you need to put the work in, and that's the truth. Don't be fooled by promises from those who only want your money. Think intelligently, work out hard and eat healthy—that's the real, and the only, weight loss mantra.

96

2 Secrets for Losing Weight Fast, Slimming and Remaining Slim – Losing Weight Made Easy!

What degree of slimness qualifies as healthy? Experts have come up with all sorts of ways to calculate a healthy individual weight—traditional weight charts, BMI (Body Mass Index) calculators, and now SBMI (Smart Body Mass Index) calculators, based on your height and weight, and age. But falling into the healthy range on the BMI and being happy when you look in the mirror are two different things. Look around at the gym, and you'll see lots of people who look great already still struggling to lose weight.

Of course, there are those lucky few who seem able to eat whatever they want without gaining an ounce. We all know a few; you've probably sat at the lunch table with them, watching them eat their chocolate bars and complain how hungry they still are, while you stare glumly down at your salad. They never have to worry about losing weight, even as they age. Most of us, however, have to work hard to reach our goal weight, and keep working to maintain it. There's no finish line; it's a never-ending process. And that's where many people fall short. How do you continue your diet plan, exercise, and have self-control indefinitely?

Mix it Up

The best method of controlling your weight is to keep switching up your routine. Add yoga a few days a week to replace a diet you're getting burned out on, with your personal trainer's sign-off, of course. Routine fatigue is one of the most dangerous opponents of weight maintenance; it creeps up on you, and so does the weight.

Stay Positive

The power of the mind is an amazing thing, and you can use it for both good and ill in your weight loss and maintenance plan. You are what you think you are most of the time, and if you allow yourself to criticize your image every time you look in the mirror, and live in constant fear of the weight you've lost returning, sooner or later, it will. This is known as a self-fulfilling prophecy, and it's a dangerous game. It's hard to look in the mirror and accept everything you see, though, so try instead to find one positive thing in your reflection to compliment yourself on. It'll take work, but you're used to work—that's how you got to your goal weight in the first place!

97

Losing Weight Quickly from Your Midriff – Follow These Simple, Mind-Blowing Tips

The belly is one of the most difficult areas to lose weight from, and also the area that makes most people want to lose weight in the first place. There are tips upon tips on the internet on how to lose that stubborn belly fat. You may have tried some, or you may have tried them all. And still, that potbelly hangs on. Give it another try with these proven tips to lose weight from your midsection.

Begin with Understanding

Understand that most of these internet tips on how to lose weight from your midsection are myths, unproven by science or seasoned experts.

Understand, too, that each article you read, each person you talk to, and every website you visit will have a different theory on losing weight fast. It's up to you to do the research and find the one that suits you best. This will take time; if you're constantly switching strategies because of a recommendation from your coworker's cousin's boyfriend, you're not going to make much progress. Settle on something, give it two or three weeks, and if you're not seeing results, *then* move on to something different.

Understand your body type: do you lose weight fast or slow? Do you have a stocky build or a longer, leaner one? Do you store weight in your hips, or your waistline? Once you know your body type, you'll be able to work out a better strategy for yourself, based on what has worked for people with similar body types and metabolisms.

Understand that any plan to lose weight will call for changes in your diet, exercise routine, and outlook. You can't have your cake and eat it, too—you should be prepared for some hard work.

A Successful Program to Lose Weight Quickly and Trim Your Belly

Several leading doctors and researchers have proven that any successful weight loss program must be a combination of three components: a regimented diet, cardiovascular exercise, and a strength and endurance building program. Ideally, this should all be done under professional guidance, by a trainer who can recommend a program customized for you. But here are some general guidelines, so you'll know a good plan when you see it.

1. Diet

Choose a diet which focuses on smaller portions eaten five or six times daily. Your body will be able to digest more efficiently, resulting in less fat storage. Two of your meals should be rich in protein, as they feed your muscles and increase your metabolism. Reduce your intake of fats and carbs as the day progresses.

2. Cardiovascular Exercise

Any program focused on trimming belly fat needs to include regular cardiovascular exercise, which helps shed pounds from all over the body, including your stomach. Try a variety of general cardio exercises, as well as exercises which target the abs. Some examples of targeted abdominal exercises include sit ups, crunches, and planks.

Remember, that belly fat is stubborn. Losing weight fast doesn't mean you'll see results overnight; it might be a while before the fat starts melting from your belly and you can see a noticeable difference.

98

How to Lose Weight Fast and Easy – Lose Weight with These 3 Amazing Techniques

There's a lot of noise out there right now about obesity and unhealthy lifestyles. Newspapers, television media and the internet are full of features and statistics on the harmful effects this epidemic has wrought in some of the most advanced societies in the world.

According to WIN, the Weight control Information Network, 68% of all adults in the United States above 20 years of age are overweight, 64% of women and 74% of men. 35.7% of all adults are considered obese, not just overweight. These are alarming statistics, since being overweight or obese is a severe risk factor for many serious and potentially fatal illnesses like high blood pressure, diabetes, and heart disease.

To a large extent, we're responsible for this state of affairs. Most of us have an easy, comfortable life style. It's not necessary to exert ourselves to survive, and processed food is readily available and packaged for our convenience. The lessons we learned in school about the importance of healthy food are a distant memory.

When it comes to exercise, well, most of us don't. There are cars and buses and trains and elevators to take us where we need to go, so why walk? Think about it; when did you last walk any distance to reach your destination?

In short, it's important to take stock of the situation before it's too late, for ourselves and our families. Here are a few tips to start:

1. Clean Out the Kitchen Cupboard

Fill a garbage bag with all those packs of chips and processed foods. From now on, your kitchen shelves and fridge space are reserved for healthy, organic, nutritious food. This means you have to change your buying behavior, too—make a vow to never buy those products again. If you don't think you can trust yourself to walk past the cookie aisle without putting something in your cart, consider using your store's pickup service, or find out if any local stores offer delivery, so you don't have to submit to temptation by browsing the aisles. It'll save you time, too!

2. Exercise Regularly

Your body needs physical exercise. If you're not fond of the gym, or simply don't have the time, just keep a treadmill in your basement or an exercise bike in front of the TV. You can start even smaller by using the stairs every day, and see how you start losing weight!

3. Drink Water

You should also start drinking at least eight to twelve glasses of water daily, to detox your system. Most of us drink endless cups of coffee, tea, or even soda at our desks, but this has to stop. Tea and coffee should be consumed in moderation; substitute every other cup with water to start, and you'll be well on your way to breaking the cycle.

99

Weight Loss Through Law of Attraction – Follow These 4 Simple Steps

Yes, you got it right—it is possible to lose weight, get back into shape and slip into that old bikini without a diet or exercise. Law of attraction, popularly explained in "The Secret," can really work wonders. But to get the full benefit, one must understand what law of attraction, positive affirmation, and manifestation is. How does the power of the mind work to generate overwhelming results, such as weight loss?

They say "like attracts like," and in this case that means you're bound to attract what you believe in. If you believe you're fat, obese, or unattractive, nature responds by making you into what you believe. If, on the other hand, you see yourself as slim, charming, and attractive, that's what you'll become. Allow the power of your thoughts to send your desired vibrations out to the universe, and the universe will respond by delivering what you believe.

You've probably heard that "thoughts become things," and this is a fact. We often concentrate on the negative aspects of a situation, and the result is depressing, frustrating feelings. The art is to think positively, even in adversity, and you'll be amazed to see the results for yourself. If you consistently tell yourself you've lost weight, it'll become true, and you'll have the last laugh.

The question then is how to use the principles of law of attraction to attain quick weight loss, and remain slim. It's not exactly simple, but it's not difficult, either. You have to tune your thinking, attitude and approach to all the elements of your life in a positive manner. Following these steps can help you attain your goals.

1. Express your gratitude for the way you are—your health, your body, your lifestyle and so on. Be thankful to the universe for having given you the ultimate gift—*you.*

2. Start loving yourself the way you are. Don't grumble about your body. Be happy, and love yourself. This brings you closer to what you're seeking.

3. Focus your thoughts on the benefits you'll reap by losing weight. Beauty, attractiveness, social appreciation, positive remarks from friends and family, and above all, inner happiness. Don't think about the hard work that needs to be put in, or the sacrifices you need to make to lose weight. These are negative thoughts; don't entertain them. Keep a positive frame of mind.

4. Finally, the most important part of applying this principle is to start believing you've already achieved your goal. Start acting as if you've already lost the weight. Imagine yourself on a sunny beach, in your old favorite bikini. Send the signal to the universe that this is what you are, and nature will mold you into your vision.

The degree of success in attaining your weight loss goals through law of attraction is entirely in your hands—or, more precisely, in your mind. There's no dietician or physical trainer to shift the blame to. If you believe in yourself, which you should, and believe in winning the game, you'll definitely lose weight.

100

Weight Loss Programs – 4 Frequently Asked Questions

Is there such a thing as permanent weight loss, or guaranteed way to lose weight and stay slim? The answer is both yes and no. A successful weight loss program only works for as long as you follow it; the weight only stays off as long as you're serious about your efforts.

A number of weight loss programs, including pills, are advertised in print media, TV, and the web, all promising instant results. "Learn how I lost ____ pounds in only a week!" In practice, none of these things work the way they're advertised. They're only a sales gimmick, a trap for innocent, naive people eager to get slim.

The weight loss industry is an evergreen, thriving machine. Globally, it's likely a billion dollar industry, though no authentic figures are available on the number of people who buy into these schemes, or the revenue generated by their desperation.

1. Do We Have True Weight Loss Programs?

The market is full of health and fitness programs. Those who are eager to lose weight and gain control need not feel discouraged; there are some genuine programs which, if followed religiously, produce amazing results, but these results are never the same for any two individuals. You can't compare yourself to someone who lost two inches or ten pounds when you've only lost one inch and five pounds. Everyone's metabolism is different; it might take you longer to achieve the same results, but try to concentrate on the progress *you* have made, instead of comparing yourself to others.

2. Are Weight Loss Programs Successful?

The success of any program, and more importantly, the degree of success you'll achieve, depends on a number of factors. They include the quality of the program, your own lifestyle habits (what you eat, how much, and how often) and the type and quantity of liquids you consume. It also depends on the nature of your work and work schedule. Is your job physically demanding, or do you work at a desk all day? Are you sitting or standing for most of the day? There are countless factors and combinations of factors, all of which will influence your results.

3. Can Diet Affect the Results of a Weight Management Program?

Absolutely! Most programs target two elements, diet and physical exercise. The results of any program can be influenced by a thorough analysis of these two factors and how they're affected by our daily diet, work, and household routine, determining where these fall short, and substituting these with a healthy diet and activities. One has to be disciplined, therefore, in following the rules and recommendations; any lapses, and you won't reach your goal.

4. Do I Need to Consult My Doctor Before Choosing a Program?

Yes, the best option is to consult your doctor before choosing a program. Your doctor knows your medical history and needs, and can make intelligent recommendations to help you reach your weight loss goals. However, doctor's visits are expensive and time consuming, so you could buy a known weight reduction program and follow it religiously in the convenience of your own home. Just be careful of what you buy.

If you're really serious about losing weight and keeping it off, carefully explore the pros and cons of various options available, and make a measured decisions. It's your body and your responsibility. You only live once!

101

Lose Weight on Vacation? You Must Be Kidding – 3 Tips on How to Avoid Post Vacation Blues!

Who doesn't go on vacation with family or friends and come back tanned and glowing? That glow might fade a bit, though, when you hear comments on the first day back at work like, "You must have enjoyed that vacation…you gained a bit of weight, didn't you?" And then you have to start your workouts again and start from scratch to lose weight.

It's natural to gain a few pounds while on vacation. We go on vacation to enjoy and and indulge in gourmet delights, lazy mornings, late-night partying and more. The extra pounds we gain in those few weeks are enough to keep us busy for the rest of the year.

But you can avoid this on your next vacation, and not have to worry about the afterglow of your trip being flattened by a silly remark from an acquaintance or your own realization in the mirror. It's easier said than done, sure, but an ounce of prevention is worth pounds of cure.

1. The Sumptuous Buffets

One of the biggest culprits in a holiday resort or cruise ship is the breakfast and lunch buffets. There's so much to choose from, it's hard not to take some of everything. That's fine, but pick up the healthy options. Fill up your plate with greens, and add a small serving of meat or cold cuts. Choose food with vitamins and minerals, avoid fatty food, carbohydrates, and processed foods—and stay away from those fries! Fill up on local fresh fruit, especially the citrus, and have a cup of green tea.

For lunch, start with another plate of greens, followed by soup and fresh whole wheat bread—sorry, no butter! You can have a small portion of lean meat with no fatty trimmings; opt for steamed fish. You'll also find a good variety of organic food, so opt for that.

2. Evening Dinners...

Evening is the hardest time to control. Dinners are often a prolonged affair with plenty of alcohol involved. Control yourself and settle for a glass of dry wine. No cocktails; they're high in calories. Desserts are also irresistible, especially at dinner. Indulge if you must, but do so in moderation. Remember, the emphasis during a vacation isn't weight loss, but weight maintenance.

A Late Stroll

A stroll after dinner is always recommended; it will, to some extent, help you burn calories and help in balancing weight, if not losing it.

Get up late, but remember to do your basic workouts to keep you slim and trim. You can increase the joy of vacation much more, if you're aware it won't end up with a heavier you.

102

Are You Making These Common Mistakes for Quick Weight Loss?

Losing weight is important, not just for aesthetic reasons, but also because it ensures a healthier life. Sadly, in an effort to achieve quick weight loss, many people take the wrong path with a few common mistakes and beliefs with no scientific backing. Do any of these sound familiar?

Mistake #1: Eating Three Square Meals a Day

One of the old cardinal rules of a weight loss diet is that you should only eat three meals a day. Sound familiar? But the truth is it doesn't really matter how many meals you have, as long as the calories add up at the end of the day. In fact, fitness and nutrition experts recommend giving up three meals a day in favor of five or six smaller meals. This boosts your metabolism and speeds your weight loss.

Mistake #2: Avoid Snacks Between Meals

We say again: calories are calories. It doesn't matter where you get them, and there's no reason to starve yourself if you're hungry. Just make sure the snacks you choose are low-cal and healthy. You can't get away with bingeing on a box of donuts or bag of chips and expect to see weight loss. Try fruit, low-cal yogurt, raw, unsalted nuts, or vegetables.

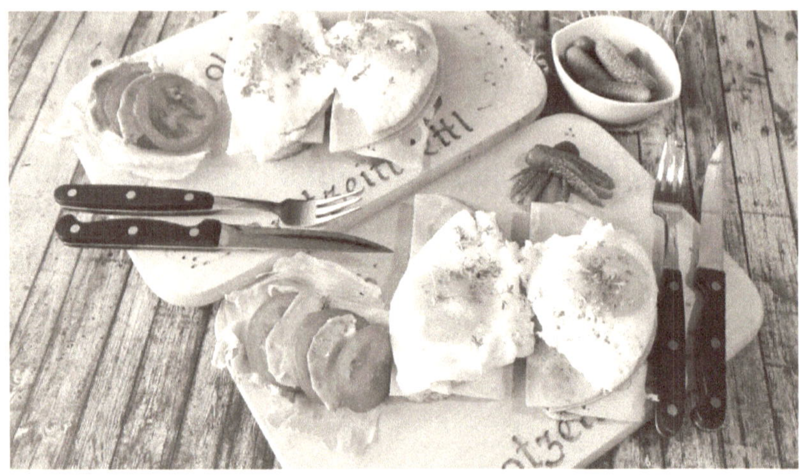

Mistake #3: Never Have Desserts

Another big mistake! Deprivation is one of the biggest reasons dieters fall off the wagon. When you deprive yourself of little pleasures, you lose motivation for your diet and have trouble sustaining it over a prolonged period of time. Dieting doesn't have to mean torturing yourself. You're allowed an occasional treat, as long as you don't overindulge. Make provision for one or two days a week when you can have your favorite dessert. You can also use it as a reward, if you've had a really good week and hit your weight loss goal.

Mistake #4: Eat All You Want – Just Exercise Regularly

This is probably only second to the "starve yourself" myth, in terms of common dieting mistakes. There must be a balance between what you put into your body and how you burn the calories. You can't have a six-course meal every two hours and expect to burn it by working out. For example, a slice of apple pie has 500 calories. To burn that off, you'd have to walk briskly for *two hours*. Keep that in mind the next time you try to tell yourself, "I'm going to the gym later…it doesn't matter what I eat now."

103

4 Ways to Lose Weight on Your Face – How to Get a Chiseled Face!

They say the face is the mirror of one's heart; I say the face is the mirror of one's health. It depicts both your state of mind and your state of body.

Additional fat on the face is the result of a generally overweight state. The face is perhaps the smallest portion of the body, and so has fewer areas like the cheeks and chin for fat to accumulate. Age is a factor, as it slows metabolism, resulting in excessive fat accumulation on the muscles, but this isn't always the case. While there's no single remedy or quick fix, there are several things you can do to slim and sculpt your face.

1. **Drink in Moderation:** Excessive intake of alcohol increases dehydration, causing water retention throughout the body, most noticeably in the face. Try to avoid alcohol whenever possible, but if you've slipped up, drink ten to twelve glasses of water daily to avoid water retention and detox the body.

2. **Exercise Regularly:** Remember that facial fat is the last to go, so don't get discouraged if you don't see results in your face right away. Remember, there's no quick fix for this; have patience. If you just can't wait, though, there are a few exercises you can do, like opening, closing, and flexing your jaws regularly. Even chewing sugar-free gum can be a good exercise for your face.

3. **Regulate Your Diet and Lifestyle:** Eat plenty of proteins and fiber; reduce carbohydrates and fat. Fill your plate with salads, boiled, steamed, and roasted vegetables, eat small meals throughout the day, and reduce salt.

The last is especially important for quick results, since salt causes water retention, particularly in the face.

4. **Yoga:** You probably already know about the fitness benefits of yoga for your body, but we highly recommend the Pranayama exercises for your face. These breathing exercises give wonderful results, and it's said they can tone all fifty-seven facial and neck muscles.

104

How to Lose Weight Fast and Easy with a Detox Diet!

You've probably heard of detox diets before, but you might not know detox can help you lose weight and burn extra belly fat. In most cases, people lose three to seven pounds in about two weeks. Before we go further, however, you need to understand the relationship between toxins in the body and being overweight. Our body gets toxins by two means; first, because of body processes, in the form of residual byproducts, and second, by consumption through air and food. These toxins are usually excreted from the body through stool or urine, but if they hang around, they can result in hormone imbalances, impaired immune system, nutritional deficiencies, and slow metabolism. The effects of toxins can be further manifested in the form of diseases such as cancer, liver disease, and cardiac problems.

The body starts gaining weight because of a slow metabolism, which stalls the fat burning process. Detoxifying our bodies at regular intervals gets rid of toxins slowing the metabolism and interfering with the body's other processes as well.

Detox Diet

A detox diet consists of fruits and vegetables, unsweetened fruit and vegetable juices, beans, lentils, oats, potatoes, brown rice, unsalted nuts, natural yogurt, olive oil, ginger, garlic, black pepper, herbal tea, fresh herbs, and fresh fish. Wherever possible, detox ingredients should be organic, to avoid consumption of further toxins; organic foods are toxin-free. One can eat these ingredients in as salad, or steamed, boiled or poached. Detox foods should only be cooked in olive oil, as other oils will add to body fat.

Foods to Avoid

Foods and beverages such as tea, coffee, red meat, chicken, sausage, salted nuts, savory snacks, butter, margarine, all white items like sugar, salt, rice, milk, cheese and cream, chocolate, jam, sweets, processed foods of any type, alcohol, and any kind of fizzy drink. The better you do at avoiding these foods during detox, the faster detox will happen.

Water, Water and More Water...

Water is the best and most natural means to detox the body. It flushes out toxins, maintains body fluid balance and, to some extent, controls appetite. You should drink about three liters of water a day for effective detox.

Weight loss requires more than physical exercise; you need determination, dedication, and motivation to live well. Detox grows on you—once you start and see the benefits for yourself, you'll likely become addicted!

105

Lose Weight in Style – How Do Celebrities Lose Weight and Keep Slim, Trim and Fit?

Ever wonder how movie stars and models maintain their perfect waistlines and lose weight in style? Why can't everyone lose weight that fast? Everyone wants a perfect, attractive body; everyone has dreamt themselves onto a poster, clad in a bikini. We wondered the same, but after a bit of research, we discovered two simple truths about how these role models lose weight.

1. Have a Powerful Incentive

Celebrities are salespeople, and their looks and body are their products. The product has to be flawless in every way, or no one wants to buy it. Celebrities know this; they know their bodies are their bread and butter and that, if they're not marketable, they'll lose their livelihood. They have no option but to lose weight, if they want to keep their jobs. You've seen it yourself; how many actresses have gained weight and fallen from the spotlight almost instantly? So, if you want to lose weight like the stars do, you need motivation as powerful as theirs. Perhaps you should be thankful you don't have as much resting on the shape of your hips as they do.

2. Have a Realistic Weight Loss Goal

One of the most discouraging things that can happen during a weight loss plan is to fail to meet your goal. There are two possible reasons for these failures; first, that you didn't try your very best, or second, the goal you set was unrealistic. Most celebrities have professional help from nutritionists or trainers, who tell them how much weight they need to lose. They don't add to these targets, once they're set; with the help of a team of experts, they work toward that single, bright goal.

You see how simple those so-called secrets of celebrities really are, so what's stopping you now? Go out and lose weight like a movie star!

The author wishes all its readers a great success in their weight loss, slimming and healthy living efforts. Remember there in nothing better in life than Wellbeing!